2-



# Weight Loss That Lasts

## Break Through the 10 Big Diet Myths

James M. Rippe, M.D.

and

Weight Watchers

WILEY

John Wiley & Sons, Inc.

Published by John Wiley & Sons, Inc., Hoboken, New Jersey
Published simultaneously in Canada

Design and composition by Navta Associates, Inc.

All photos were provided by Weight Watchers.



*Library of Congress Cataloging-in-Publication Data*

Rippe, James M.
Weight watchers weight loss that lasts : break through the 10 big diet myths / James M. Rippe.
p. cm.
Includes bibliographical references and index.
ISBN 0-471-70528-4 (cloth)
ISBN 0-471-72172-7 (pbk.)
1. Weight loss. 2. Medical misconceptions. I. Weight Watchers International. II. Title.
RM222.2.R5524 2005
613.2′5—dc22
2004023808

Printed in the United States of America

10 9 8 7 6 5 4 3 2 1

To Stephanie, Hart, Jaelin, Devon, and Jamie Rippe—
who make it all worthwhile.

JMR

To Jean Nidetch, founder of
Weight Watchers International, Inc.

KMK

# Contents

# Preface

## A personal message from James M. Rippe, M.D.

I am a cardiologist—a physician who specializes in the prevention and medical treatment of heart disease. I have spent the past twenty-five years fully engaged in the battle to lower the likelihood of heart disease for my patients and my country. In addition to my work with patients, I have written several cardiology textbooks and continue to edit the major intensive care textbook in the country, *Irwin and Rippe's Intensive Care Medicine.* I have also written books for the general public concerning simple steps that we can all take to lower our risk of heart disease. Most recently, my book *Heart Disease for Dummies* provided commonsense advice about how to lower the risk of developing heart disease or how to treat it if you already have it.

I am also a researcher. Based on my early research on the health benefits of walking, I have been called the father of the modern walking movement, an accolade of which I am extremely proud. I founded and currently direct the Rippe Lifestyle Institute (RLI) based in Massachusetts and Florida, one of the largest exercise, nutrition, and weight management research organizations in the United States. RLI's research is designed to help people understand how their diet, level of physical activity, and weight management techniques have a profound impact on both their short- and long-term health and on their quality of life. At RLI, we have studied many different aspects of weight management and have been able to observe what works and what does not work on thousands of patients. Over the last twenty years, RLI has studied thousands of people and presented hundreds of research papers at important medical and scientific meetings around the world.

Why is a cardiologist coauthoring a book on weight loss? The answer is simple: Being overweight or obese significantly increases the likelihood that you will develop heart disease—the number one killer of both men and women in the United States. Unless we make strides to help individuals control their weight, we will never get the epidemic of heart disease under control in our country, or, indeed, throughout the industrialized world.

I am not a diet doctor. It is not my purpose to convince you to follow a weight-loss plan that I developed. Instead, I am sharing with you published research on the health aspects of various methods to weight loss and helping you interpret the research so that you can make use of them in your life.

## My Collaboration with Weight Watchers

Although this is the first book that I've coauthored with Weight Watchers, we have been collaborators for more than a decade. I was introduced to Karen Miller-Kovach, currently Chief Scientific Officer at Weight Watchers, through mutual contacts. Weight Watchers was interested in putting its program through a rigorous clinical trial, and as a researcher I was interested in the opportunity to objectively study this weight-loss method. I published the findings from that study, which you'll learn more about in this book.

Karen and I have maintained our collaborative relationship over the years. We've shared the podium at speaking engagements, discussed the latest weight-loss research, and swapped greeting cards over the holidays. It is a pleasure to be collaborating with her on this important book.

I am proud to be associated with Weight Watchers because the organization focuses on two things that are extremely important to me. First, Weight Watchers is committed to developing programs, products, and services that promote healthy, sustainable weight loss. Second, the Weight Watchers program is based completely on sound science. Weight Watchers has scientific data to demonstrate its track record in helping people achieve long-term weight loss. In forty-plus years, Weight Watchers has evolved into the most trusted name in weight management—one that educates people based on scientific developments and real-life experiences in sustaining weight loss.

The Weight Watchers program makes sense because it combines the findings from two types of equally important laboratories: scientific research laboratories and real-life laboratories. Weight Watchers is an active participant in the global forum of diverse disciplines related to weight management—everything from cardiology to psychology. The organization synthesizes the learnings from ongoing medical and scientific research and turns them into practical reality. This involves constant in-field testing and adaptation of their program. The experience of helping millions of people through Weight Watchers meetings also provides a living laboratory for observing what is necessary to achieve sustainable weight loss. The science is only useful if it fills a need and can be applied in real life.

The result is the experience at Weight Watchers meetings. They provide coaching and real-life insights so that participants can make the positive changes required to lose weight and keep it off. Participants learn that there are different paths to losing weight, but all involve making wise food choices, being physically active, having a positive mindset, and living in a supportive atmosphere. Weight Watchers is a realistic way of life for sustainable weight loss.

Weight Watchers has the only structured program with a legitimate ongoing database of individuals who have successfully lost weight and kept it off. The Weight Watchers organization has graciously allowed me access to this database and these individuals—the first time that an academic researcher has ever been granted ongoing access to this important body of information. In this book, we will share with you the inspirational stories of several individuals from the database.

Weight Watchers and I share the same goal: to provide you with sound, sensible, scientifically based information so that you can make informed decisions about losing and managing your weight in a healthy and satisfying way. We strive to help you deal with the modern challenges of society, where food is too plentiful, food choices are laden with calories, and food advertising is everywhere. This abundant environment, coupled with our society's dramatic decrease in physical activity brought about by technological advances like garage door openers, remote controls, and even cars, creates a combustible mix. Weight gain is guaranteed in a society that has too many calories being consumed and too few calories being spent.

## My Personal Story of Achieving Sustainable Weight Loss

To look at me as a slim and fit man, you might wonder how I could ever understand the challenges of losing weight. Through my personal experience with being overweight, I do understand. Like many of you, there have been a few times in my life when I have gained substantial amounts of weight. Let me tell you a little bit about my personal journey to sustainable weight loss.

My first experience with weight gain came during my first two years of college. I entered college at the relatively trim size of 5'9" and 154 pounds. As a child and in my teen years, I participated in numerous sports programs and had a very active lifestyle. When I got to college, it was a different story. I stopped playing sports, and I was overwhelmed by the amount of food that was available on the cafeteria-style eating plan. The arrangement seemed too good to resist! I routinely filled my entire tray with food and thought nothing of going back for second or third helpings. Now that I look back on it, the result was entirely predictable: I gained weight. Toward the end of my sophomore year, I looked in the mirror and suddenly realized that the guy looking back at me was pudgy. I had been ignoring my weight gain for so long that it took a while for me to admit that I needed to lose weight.

My second bout of adult weight gain was very intense. During my medical internship and residency, I was required to spend one out of every three nights awake taking care of desperately sick patients. To help doctors get through the night, the hospital provided "the midnight meal." I often consumed a complete dinner between 11:00 P.M. and midnight, after having eaten my first dinner earlier in the evening. Once again, the result was predictable. During this two-year period, my weight ballooned.

Many of you will be able to relate to my third battle with weight gain. It occurred after a happy event in my life—my marriage. I married a wonderful woman who is a very good cook. Gradually, over the first three or four years of our marriage, I once again gained weight. Believe it or not, it took a trip through my own Rippe Health Assessment at Florida Hospital Celebration Health to discover the consequences of my happy lifestyle. Not only had my weight gone up but my fitness level had declined by 20% and my cholesterol level had nearly doubled. As a cardiologist, I knew this was not good!

As I look back at these three periods of adult weight gain, I realize that like so many people, I had deluded myself with a number of myths. The first myth I relied on was that because I was an active person, I could eat anything I wanted and not worry about weight gain. I also convinced myself that a little weight gain would not harm my health. I fell prey to the myth that just by exercising alone I could somehow melt away the extra pounds.

To get beyond the myths, I trained myself to think about each one, find the kernel of truth and discard the rest, then take positive actions to lose the weight and keep it off. I am proud to tell you that I am now back down to my high school weight. I know that the key to maintaining that weight is to be honest with myself and take those daily steps toward sustainable weight loss that have worked for me and hundreds of my patients.

As my personal experience and years as a physician have taught me, a solid understanding of what you can do in your daily life is important to achieve lasting weight loss. I am convinced that this book can help you do just that. This worthy challenge was significant enough to bring me together with the leading company in the area of healthy weight management. Weight Watchers and I share the same vision: to offer you insights, observations, and experience so that you can lose weight for good.

# Acknowledgments

First, we would like to thank the Weight Watchers Lifetime Members whose weight-loss success inspires us each day. Special thanks to those members who shared their personal stories in this book. Their personal triumphs provided valuable insight into what it takes to achieve sustainable weight loss in the real world. We hope you find their stories as inspiring and informative as we have.

We are indebted to the scientists who have contributed to the science of weight management over the years. Their hard work is the foundation of this book. We also want to acknowledge Drs. Rena Wing and James Hill, who founded the National Weight Control Registry over a decade ago. We have gained valuable insights from them and quote numerous findings from the registry.

We would like to thank all our colleagues at Weight Watchers International, Inc., and the Rippe Lifestyle Institute. Particular appreciation goes to Beth Porcaro Grady, who manages Dr. Rippe's book projects, and to Carol Moreau, who keeps his work life in order and moving forward. We are indebted to the hard work and tireless efforts of Mindy Hermann and Evren Bilimer, who helped turn this book from a kernel of an idea into a reality, as well as to that of our editor, Tom Miller, for his invaluable suggestions.

James M. Rippe, M.D.
Karen Miller-Kovach, M.S., R.D.

# Introduction

# The truth will set you free

Wouldn't you do just about anything to learn the secret for losing weight and keeping it off? You're not alone. Millions of people are overweight and trying to lose weight. But if you're like a lot of the people we advise every day, you're also tired and frustrated with everything you hear and read about dieting. You don't need health care professionals to convince you that losing weight is important. But as health care professionals, we can show you the path to sustainable weight loss by taking you behind the curtain of the science so that you can break through the myths that may be holding you back.

## Sustainable Weight Loss Is Possible

The thought of losing weight can be daunting. Wouldn't it be great if someone could wave a magic wand over your head and make those extra pounds disappear? But that is not possible. Losing weight takes time and effort. That's particularly true if you don't have the right method, approaches, and encouragement to help you along.

We're here to give you good news: Sustainable weight loss is not hidden in the lost continent of Atlantis. It is not a myth. With the right directions and an accurate roadmap, it is possible to avoid the false turns that are so common. Having been there ourselves, we can tell you that you can even enjoy the experience. The key is to be armed with the facts, to be able to separate the weight-loss truths from the big diet myths. With a solid foundation, it is possible to tackle any challenge and avoid any future traps that may come your way. Our goal is to present you with the science behind the myths that you hear every day, then help you interpret how you can make that science work for you.

## Myths and Weight Loss

Myths are a part of every society and culture. They help explain common experiences that are mysterious, frightening, or difficult to understand. Ancient civilizations used myths to explain aspects of the world that they could not comprehend. Joseph Campbell, author of the book *The Power of Myth,* explains that we need myths to survive and to explain and understand our existence.

Myths *are* powerful. They can inspire us to great heights. But they can also become traps when they mask the full truth. If you go beyond the kernel of truth that forms the basis of the myth and believe that every aspect of the myth is true, you can become paralyzed into inaction because the myth seemingly explains everything.

Many popular weight-loss methods can be attractive and persuasive. Who hasn't tried at least a few of the latest and greatest weight-loss plans? These methods are appealing because they are based on a believable myth, a convincing scientific explanation, and a fantastic promise: the pitch is that if you buy into the myth, you will lose weight quickly.

Perhaps you believed the myth that simply by cutting back on fat you could lose weight permanently. Maybe you believed the myth that cutting out most carbohydrates would magically melt away your extra fat and pounds. Perhaps you subscribed to the common myth that if you simply began exercising more, your weight would come off. We wish we could tell you that these myths were true. While each has some kernels of truth, they're missing quite a bit as well. That's the point of this book; we'll fill you in on the whole story.

Myths have the power to keep you riding the weight-loss roller coaster or prevent you from trying again. That is why it is so important to pull out the kernel of truth and discard the rest. Until you separate the truth from the myth, you won't achieve your goal of sustainable weight loss.

Stop in your local bookstore, browse online, or watch one of television's morning shows and you will quickly see that weight-loss myths are abundant. One popular myth states that carrying a few extra pounds around doesn't really have an impact on your health. The myth has a kernel of truth: carrying around a few extra pounds is not as risky as carrying around a lot of extra pounds. But the whole truth is that even gaining small amounts of weight as the years go by carries a health risk.

Today, an even more widespread but fading myth is that a low-carbohydrate diet magically melts away pounds and is *the* answer to weight loss. Once again, there is an element of truth to this myth. Many people eat overly large portions of carbohydrates like pasta and bread, as well as too many foods with added sugars and highly processed flour. This type of eating can contribute to weight gain in very significant ways. Furthermore, carbohydrate foods supply a majority of our calories. So cutting back on empty calories from added sugar and highly processed flour can help you lose weight as long as you don't fill your diet with low-carbohydrate, calorie-rich foods.

Or what about the common myth that all you need to do is go to the gym and work out to lose weight? There is a kernel of truth to the relationship between regular exercise and weight loss. But individuals who think that they can lose weight simply by increasing their exercise program and not controlling their food intake are almost always embarking on a futile journey.

We all have myths. Some are wonderful because they inspire us. Some get in the way of our progress. Myths can be busted through knowledge. The road to sustainable weight loss begins when you get rid of the weight-loss myths standing in your way and learn how to make the science of weight loss work for you.

This book is about weight-loss truths. Our goal is to tell you the whole truth about how you can lose weight for good. In doing so, we can help you base your weight-loss efforts on solid principles that work and that are based on years of experience and hundreds of scientific studies, many of which were performed at the Rippe Lifestyle Institute (RLI) or with people following the Weight Watchers program. Together, we've had the opportunity to learn from countless people about what works when it comes to sustainable weight loss. We know that with the right method, long-term weight loss is possible.

## Meet Those Who Won by Losing

When it comes to weight loss, you probably have your own myths. We believe that we've heard most of them. Some people talk to us about their belief in extreme diets that cut out entire food groups. Some tell us that their big bones, menopause, work schedule, or some other reason makes weight loss impossible. Some are sure that all it will take is a bit more exercise to lose the weight. Throughout this book, we will share with you the insights of successful Weight Watchers members who believed in these myths and tell you their stories of how they triumphed over the myths and achieved sustainable weight loss.

Millions of people have learned how to achieve sustainable weight loss through Weight Watchers. They won by losing, and you can profit from their experience. Use their stories as a source of information and motivation for yourself. In this book, you will meet a wide variety of people, including Sandra Franczyk, whose weight went down and up many times as she believed in several weight-loss myths before losing weight for good. You will read the success story of Rebecca Hill, who denied that she had a weight problem until her husband got so frustrated with her weight and eating habits that he packed her suitcase and threatened to send her to a "fitness farm." You will be introduced to two people with lifelong severe asthma who didn't realize that their weight was making their asthma worse. As they lost weight, their asthma improved dramatically.

This book presents the ten big diet myths that are sizable barriers to sustainable weight loss. Let's look carefully at the myths; you may find that you believed in them. We will explore the kernels of truth behind each myth, then give you the whole truth so that you can turn it into a powerful agent of sustainable weight loss. Unravel the myths and lose the weight. Even better, once you understand them, you will be positioned to spot future myths and avoid being lured into their trap. This book will arm you with the knowledge you need to finally lose that weight for good!

## How to Use This Book

- Early in each of the book's next ten chapters, we include a myth.
- Each myth is based on kernels of truth, so each chapter explores the kernels and the power behind the myth.
- The chapter then goes on to take you from the kernels of truth to the whole truth—giving you the background on where the kernels came from, exposing pieces of the myth that are not true, and summarizing the science about the myth.
- Throughout each chapter, you will read about the personal triumphs of people just like you who were able to seek out and use the kernel of truth in a myth to reach their weight goals.
- Each chapter concludes with an action plan to give you some steps to get started. By understanding the scientific research and evidence that supports or discredits the myths, you'll have the knowledge to make sound decisions.

## Our Mission

We hope that as you join us in reading this book, you can profit from both the scientific literature and the insights of others to reach your own weight-loss goals. We believe that the knowledge you will gain will put you on the path to sustainable weight loss.

Enjoy the ride! In this book, we will help you find the truth that will set you free.

# Chapter 1

# Is sustainable weight loss possible?

Chances are, you've heard the same statistic over and over again. And if it's true that 95% of diets end in failure, it's reasonable to conclude that trying to lose weight is not worth the effort. Nobody is going to tell you that it is easy to achieve weight loss that lasts. But it is possible. Let's begin to explore exactly how to win the weight-loss battle.

# Myth 1 You can't lose weight and keep it off

*Believers Beware!*

The sad reality is that you have about as great a chance of losing weight and keeping it off as you do of winning the lottery. This is just a simple fact of life. Everybody knows it. Every magazine article and television show on the topic gives the same facts: 95% of diets fail, and for those who do lose weight, it's just about guaranteed that they'll gain it all back. When the media interviews experts who study weight loss for a living, they all say this is true.

The results of weight-loss failure surround us. Everybody has coworkers, neighbors, friends, and family who have lost weight—lots of it—only to gain it back within a relatively short period of time.

There are many reasons why sustained weight loss is impossible. For some people, it is because they have a medical condition like a slow thyroid or a naturally slow metabolism. Another reason is that losing weight slows down the metabolism, forcing your body to regain the weight even though you're eating less.

Losing weight and keeping it off? It's just not possible!

## Kernels of Truth

There are reports from credible sources that give some pretty negative statistics. In the 1950s, Dr. Albert J. Stunkard summarized his findings about weight-loss methods available at that time. The finding was that 95% of diets fail. Likewise, an expert panel from the National Institutes of Health (NIH) reported in 1992 that people who completed a weight-loss program could expect to regain about two-thirds of the loss after one year and virtually all their lost weight after five years. These two reports are widely used and reused in the media and in scientific circles.

Another kernel of truth is that no single weight-loss method available today can help every overweight or obese person get down to an ideal weight and stay there forever. This book shows that that there is no one-size-fits-all approach to weight loss. Every person needs a slightly different approach.

It's also true that weight loss means a lower metabolism—the number of calories burned in the course of daily living. You'll read more about metabolism in the following chapters, but it's based on the fact that a smaller body simply needs fewer calories than a larger body. A smaller body typically has less muscle on it, and this translates into a lower metabolism. In addition, restricting calories during the weight-loss process can cause metabolism to slow down a bit, especially if the restriction is extreme (for example, an 800-calorie-a-day diet). The effect isn't enough to prevent weight loss, but it will slow down the rate of loss.

And it's also true that certain medical conditions and treatments can make weight loss more difficult. A slow thyroid, called *hypothyroidism*, slows metabolism and calorie burning. Medications, such as steroids used to treat inflammatory diseases, several drugs used to treat anxiety, depression, and similar conditions, and some drugs used to treat diabetes, stimulate the appetite. For people taking these medications, it's tough to stay committed to a weight-loss program because they are truly hungry.

Finally, our environment works against sustained weight loss. We are surrounded by a lot of food that is filled with calories, tastes good,

*Have you ever heard . . .*

**"Since I can't keep weight off, I'm better off just accepting myself the way I am at my current weight."**

Excess weight increases your disease risk. We discuss this in detail in the next chapter. Although positive self-reinforcement is important, losing weight and keeping it off is paramount for your health. This book provides you with the proof—both from the world of science and from experiences of Weight Watchers members—that sustainable weight loss is possible.

and is heavily advertised. We also live in an environment where modern technology has taken away a lot of our opportunities to burn calories. We don't even have to get up from the couch to change the channels on our televisions anymore. The combination of the two—too much great-tasting food and too little activity—can make sustained weight loss a challenge.

## The Whole Truth

### The Old Numbers Don't Tell the Full Story

The reports about diet failure need to be put into context. The discouraging 95% statistic dates back to the 1950s. Dr. Stunkard, the father of that number, is the first to say that it is no longer accurate because weight-loss methods today are so different from those used fifty years ago. Moreover, most weight-loss studies clump all dieting methods into a single pool (as if the Cabbage Soup Diet and a doctor-supervised medical program were the same) and are based on a one-time effort. Finally, the typical person who enrolls in a clinical study at the obesity clinic of a research university is not a typical American who wants to lose weight.

To get a more accurate picture of the incidence of sustained weight loss, a group of researchers randomly polled people from the general

# Personal Triumph

**Sandra Franczyk**
ILLINOIS

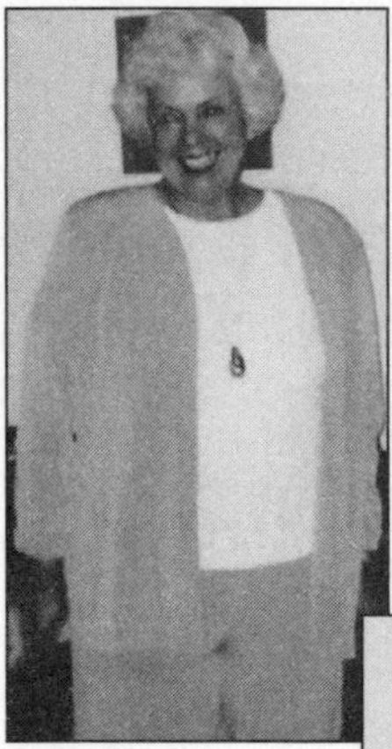

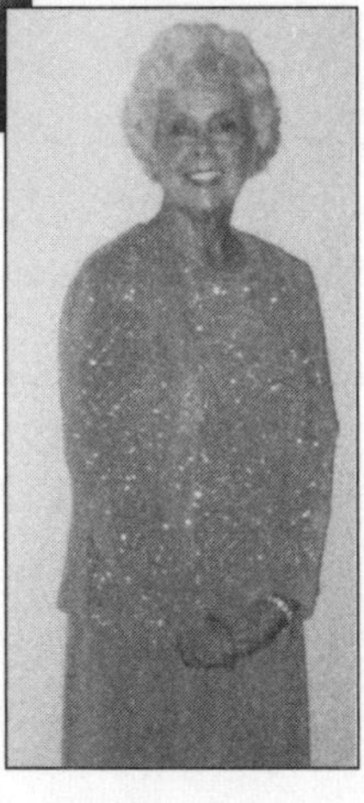

*"I don't intend to ever go back to my old habits. Those days are gone."*

Sandra Franczyk battled her weight for a good part of her adult life, having lost weight many times only to gain it back. She tried a storefront weight-loss center and numerous other approaches but was unable to achieve the lasting weight loss that she so wanted. Then she joined Weight Watchers and gained a new perspective on managing her weight. Sandra left behind the many weight-loss myths she had once believed in.

By incorporating the weight-loss success factors that are built into the Weight Watchers program, Sandra kept weight off for the first time in her life. "I closely monitor what I eat. In restaurants, I don't just order what is on the menu. I ask questions about foods I might want to order. I never was very active, but once I joined Weight Watchers, I started to exercise. Now I walk or use the exercise bike at least one hour per day. Now that I've been so successful, I don't intend to ever go back to my old habits. Those days are gone."

Sandra lost 49 pounds to reach her goal.

public and asked them about their weight-loss experiences. More than one-half of five hundred people surveyed had lost at least 10% of their maximal body weight at some point in their adult life (there will be more on the health benefits of a 10% weight loss in chapter 2). Among those who had intentionally lost weight, almost 50% reported having kept it off for at least one year at the time of the survey, and 25% stated that it had been at least five years. The researchers concluded that sustainable weight loss is not nearly as uncommon as we've been led to believe.

In a different study, a team of researchers from Drexel University surveyed Weight Watchers members who reached their goal and completed the six-week maintenance program. That survey of more than one thousand people found that an average of more than three-fourths of the weight that was lost was still gone after one year and almost one-half after five years. This contrasts sharply with the 1992 NIH report that people who complete a weight-loss program can expect to keep off one-third of the loss after one year and virtually none at five years. The Weight Watchers data were presented at a 2004 international conference on obesity, causing quite a stir. Obesity experts attributed the superior results to the combination of healthy food choices, regular physical activity, positive behavior changes, and supportive atmosphere that are all an integral part of the Weight Watchers program.

## Incorporate Success Factors into Your Weight-Loss Method

How you lose weight makes a difference in how much you lose and how successful you are in keeping it off. In 1995, the Institute of Medicine (IOM), a nonprofit organization whose mission is to advise U.S. policy makers on health-related issues in an unbiased and science-based way, issued a report about weight loss. The IOM's *Weighing the Options* report evaluated the pool of weight-loss research and included a summary of those factors with proven links to weight-loss success. The more success factors you make part of your weight-loss method, the more likely you are to win. All of these success factors have been incorporated into the Weight Watchers program (see the Afterword for more about this).

**RESEARCH-BACKED FACTORS PREDICTING WEIGHT-LOSS SUCCESS**

| Factors Linked with Reaching a Weight-Loss Goal | Factors Linked with Sustainable Weight Loss |
|---|---|
| Attendance at a program | Regular physical activity |
| Weight loss early in the program | Self-monitoring weight and food-related behavior |
| Sticking with it | Positive coping skills |
| Social support | Keeping in contact with people who helped with weight loss |
| Regular physical activity | "Normal" eating patterns |
| Behavior modification techniques | Health improvements |
| Self-monitoring | |
| Goal setting | |

*Source:* Adapted from Institute of Medicine. *Weighing the Options. Criteria for Evaluating Weight-Management Programs.* Washington, D.C.: National Academy Press, 1995.

## Sustainable Weight Loss Is Possible

In addition to the inspiring stories throughout this book, there are two large databases filled with evidence that sustainable weight loss *is* possible: the National Weight Control Registry (NWCR) and the Lifetime Member (LTM) Database from Weight Watchers. These two databases include information on thousands of people like you, your friends, and your family members who have successfully lost weight and kept it off.

Over a decade ago, Drs. Rena Wing and James Hill founded the NWCR, which includes several thousand people who have lost at least 30 pounds and kept the weight off for at least one year. As of 2003, NWCR participants had lost an average of 66 pounds and kept it off for an average of five years.

The Weight Watchers LTM Database is the largest and longest-standing database on people who have successfully lost weight. Any Weight Watchers member who reaches a goal weight that is within the healthy range and maintains that weight through a six-week maintenance phase of the Program is included in the LTM Database. The two databases have some overlap because there are people in the

LTM Database who have also volunteered their information to NWCR.

*Have you ever heard . . .*

**"Since I am doomed to fail at sustaining at my weight loss, why even try?"**

With all the success factors of sustainable weight loss in place, trying is *very* important. If you have followed an extreme diet in the past, you know that weight loss is doable and so is regaining weight. The best strategy is to look for a comprehensive weight-loss method, then make it work for you.

How did the people who are part of the NWCR and Weight Watchers LTM Database succeed? They simply learned how to incorporate the basics of a comprehensive weight-loss method into their lives using approaches that work for them. As you will learn, the habits and skills that they developed as part of the weight-loss process have become so second nature that they say sustaining the loss is easier than taking the weight off in the first place!

These basic components are so important that they are a common thread throughout this book. They have also spawned their own myths and traps. By looking at the remaining nine myths more closely, you'll be able to avoid the traps that may be getting in the way of your successful weight loss.

In order to overcome the powerful myth that it is not possible to sustain weight loss, you need to have all four components in place: making wise food choices, being physically active, making positive lifestyle changes, and creating a supportive atmosphere. Let's look more closely at each one.

## Make Wise Food Choices

Our food world is complicated. We are surrounded by tasty, affordable food choices. We are constantly reminded of food by the media,

**How They Do It**

Basic Components in a Comprehensive Weight-Loss Method

- Wise food choices
- Regular physical activity
- Positive lifestyle change
- Supportive atmosphere

advertisements, and the presence of restaurants and fast-food places everywhere. Making wise food choices is a vital skill. People who adopt specific strategies to deal with food choices are well on their way to sustainable weight loss.

This may take a bit of thinking ahead. It may seem obvious, but many people neglect this important success factor. We're not referring to detailed planning, which is not possible for most of us because of our hectic schedules. Thinking ahead means that you

1. Always have foods available that you want to eat
2. Have access to fresh fruits and vegetables
3. Start the day with a good healthy breakfast
4. Plan healthy snacks
5. Plus dozens of other simple actions to make wise food choices

Finding the eating structure that fits you best helps you create a livable, sustainable eating plan to match your food preferences. It's important to enjoy the food and the eating patterns you use to lose weight because these are the same foods and patterns that will help you keep the weight off.

## Include Regular Physical Activity

An overwhelming majority of the NWCR volunteers are physically active virtually every day. People who have sustained weight loss have figured out how to incorporate regular physical activity into their lives. The most popular activity is one that is easy for almost all of us to do—walking. People who successfully sustain their weight loss get so much benefit from regular physical activity that they wouldn't dream of a day without it.

Regular physical activity has three important elements. The first is that the activity has to fit into your life, whether in a set block of time or in little nooks and crannies throughout the day. You can squeeze in a bit of activity by taking the stairs at work, parking farther away from the store on errands, taking a ten-minute walk at lunchtime, or walking the dog at the end of the day.

These activities may sound too small to make a difference. But if you take a daily ten-minute walk at lunchtime for a year and change nothing else about your eating or activity, you can lose more than five pounds! Imagine the result if you incorporated a number of these simple activities into your daily routine.

Chapter 4 presents more information about the role of exercise and strategies to incorporate it into your daily life. Throughout the book, we're hoping to show you that small lifestyle changes can translate into big changes in your weight. These positive changes are the key to sustainable weight loss.

The second element of regular physical activity may seem obvious. Find physical activities that you enjoy. If you like an activity, you're more likely to stick with it. What is right for you might be different from what works for your family members or friends. That is okay. The key is to find something that you look forward to and enjoy such as walking outdoors or doing more structured activities like swimming, bicycling, or aerobics with a favorite exercise tape. Don't turn your life upside down—your chances of success are greater if you create a plan that is livable for you.

The third element is to look for activities that you can do almost every day. Consistent exercisers get the most benefit, and once you incorporate exercise into your daily life, it becomes second nature.

## Make Positive Lifestyle Changes

The value of a positive mindset for lasting weight loss is frequently overlooked. It shouldn't be. You have to believe that you can do it—that you can lose weight and keep it off. Whether weight has become an issue only recently or if you have been overweight for a long time, having a positive mindset and making the changes that go with it are vital in accomplishing your goal of lasting weight loss.

For many of the people who share their stories in this book, their battle with the bulge was longstanding. The same holds true with the NWCR volunteers, with almost half reporting that their weight issues began in childhood. Despite this, they were able to look beyond what didn't work in the past and focus on what they wanted to achieve.

You should have both short-term and long-term goals. Short-term goals like losing weight for a special event are easier to achieve and have immediate rewards. But setting only short-term goals is not enough. You also need a long-term mindset that takes life beyond weight loss into account.

Making positive changes to your lifestyle also means taking personal responsibility for your weight. All of us have the ability to harness our internal power to make wise choices for healthy, livable, sustainable weight loss.

Lifestyle change requires focus. Both the Weight Watchers LTM Database and NWCR participants maintain a consistent focus on their weight management strategies. This does not mean that they are overly rigid with their diet or take exercise to extremes. Rather, they have learned the skill of flexible restraint and have developed habits, routines, and approaches that support their ability to sustain weight loss.

## Create a Supportive Atmosphere

A supportive atmosphere is important for losing weight and keeping it off. Eating can be a highly social event, whether during family meals, meals with friends, or in times of celebration or sorrow. The fact is that food is one of the great pleasures of life. Sharing weight goals with others helps enlist their support. It is generally much better to let people who care about you know that you are trying to control your weight. They can be of great help. There's more on this important topic in chapter 10.

# Personal Triumph

**Michele Pollack**
CALIFORNIA

Michele Pollack, a teacher, had been a Weight Watchers member at the elementary school where she teaches but stopped attending when the school year ended. Three years later, Michele returned to Weight Watchers with a girlfriend. She was recently engaged but didn't join Weight Watchers just because she was getting married—she joined because going to Weight Watchers meetings was the same as getting together with friends.

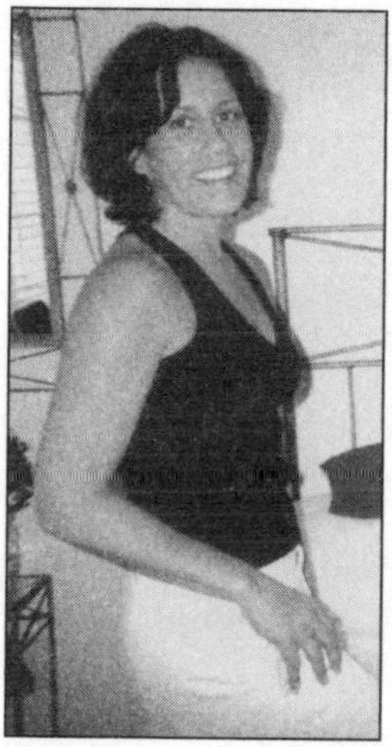

"This time, I was really motivated. I saw results right away, and going with a friend was key because we had a standing date each week. I knew I would lose the weight, and that's easy. When I reach my goal, that's when the work comes in.

*"I was not just trying to maintain, I was trying to change my lifestyle."*

"I was afraid of gaining it back because I had lost weight before and always gained it back. But I realized that I had to think about my weight every day and keep my life changes in the forefront. I was not just trying to maintain, I was trying to change my lifestyle."

Michele lost 15 pounds to reach her goal.

A study published in the *Journal of the American Medical Association* showed that the number of Weight Watchers meetings a person attended was highly predictive of total weight loss. In fact, those who attended more than 80% of meetings held during the two-year study lost more than twice as much weight as people who attended less regularly. The reason for this is simple: spending time with and learning from the experiences of others who are also losing weight is very important to accomplishing weight goals.

## Setting Unreasonable Goals Backfires

If you start out with an expectation of permanent perfection or with a weight-loss goal that is too high, you are likely to be disappointed. At the beginning of a study done at the University of Pennsylvania, participants were asked how they would feel about losing the amount of weight that the researchers could predict would be the likely result. Participants said that they would be disappointed. To be satisfied or "happy" about their weight loss, the participants said that the amount would have to be substantially more. Being dissatisfied with a realistic weight loss is counterproductive.

So what is a realistic goal? Successful weight loss is typically losing about 10% of body weight in six months. More rapid or dramatic loss is possible, but it is the exception, not the rule. For sustainable weight loss, changes should be made in a stepwise, realistic, achievable way.

## There Is No Set Point That Prevents Sustained Weight Loss

Metabolism slows down a bit during weight loss. As a result, the number of calories that the body burns during weight loss is a little bit lower than would be the case if body weight were stable. Several preliminary studies on weight loss and metabolism suggested that this dip in metabolism was permanent. In turn, these studies were used as proof that a body has a natural set point, or a body weight that it must defend. By maintaining a reduced metabolism following weight loss, the body would be more likely to regain weight, returning to its set point.

As sometimes happens in science, however, the findings from the preliminary studies did not stand up to the test of rigorous scientific scrutiny. Since those early reports, a series of precise studies using sophisticated technology have been done at the University of Alabama in Birmingham, which have proven that the set point theory is not true. Researchers showed that metabolism goes back to expected levels with sustained weight loss, confirming that metabolism and the number of calories burned during a day is related to weight and amount of muscle but not to weight loss.

## The Bottom Line

There are clearly plenty of people who have achieved sustainable weight loss. What sets them apart is not who they are but the fact that they have learned the basic components of a comprehensive weight-loss method and have incorporated them into their daily lives. They make wise food choices, are physically active, have a healthy lifestyle with a positive mindset, and are in a supportive environment.

The longer the weight loss is sustained, the easier it becomes. Success breeds success, so set yourself up for success by choosing realistic goals that are important to you and believing that you can achieve them.

The method you use to lose weight—both for taking the weight off and for keeping it off—makes a difference in how successful you will be. You are not destined to regain weight once you've lost it.

It is important to recognize the kernel of truth in the myth of sustainable weight loss. Sustainable weight loss doesn't automatically happen. You need to put your mind to it and arm yourself with the right tools. But it's time to avoid being trapped by the myth that sustainable weight loss is impossible. This entire book is based on the scientific evidence that you can achieve a lasting weight loss!

# Personal Triumph

## Kelly Hackworth Smith

TEXAS

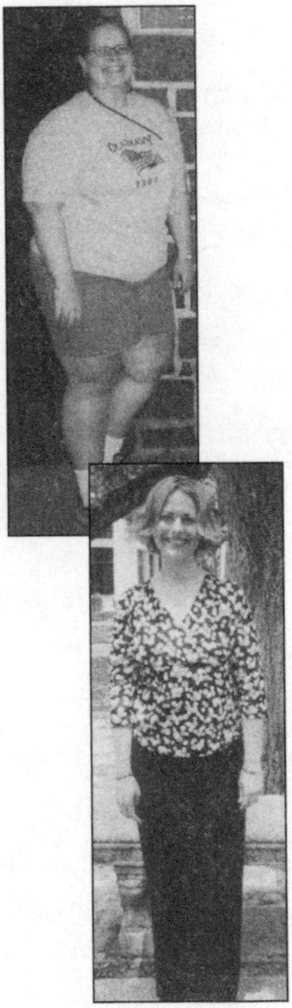

*“I had to find a way to live with food, and Weight Watchers taught me how to eat again.”*

Kelly Hackworth Smith wanted to start a family. At 273 pounds, however, Kelly was informed by her doctor that she should not try to get pregnant because pregnancy was too risky for her health and for an unborn baby.

“At my high weight, I was on a path to a lot of health problems and risks. I was only 25, and it was really frightening. My weight got out of control in college. My husband and I went out to eat a lot, and I am a stress eater.

“I had to find a way to live with food, and Weight Watchers taught me how to eat again. My Meeting Leader also helped me set smaller weight-loss goals of 25 pounds. Reaching 25 pounds was easy, but getting to 50 pounds was more challenging because I got stuck at a plateau and started sabotaging my eating and weight loss. Once I realized what I was doing, I got back on track. I got stuck again around my 75-pound and 100-pound goals.

“Looking back, I realize that I felt a lot of pressure trying to reach the higher milestones. I was trying so hard to do everything right. I also realized that I didn’t have to be perfect all the time as long as I got right back on track.”

Kelly eventually lost over 117 pounds to reach her goal weight.

## Weight Loss That Lasts

# Action Steps

The path to sustainable weight loss needs a beginning. As you put your new knowledge to work and embark on a comprehensive weight-loss method, there are several things you can do. The goal is to maximize your knowledge so that you are prepared to make informed decisions for your best approach.

- Consult with your doctor before starting any weight management program. It is a good idea to get a complete physical before beginning a diet and/or exercise program to rule out medical limitations.
- Ask your doctor or pharmacist if any of the medications that you're taking might affect your weight-loss success by increasing your appetite or slowing your metabolism. The good news is that in almost all cases other drugs are available that treat the same condition but do not affect weight. It is worth finding out whether a simple change in your medication can remove this potential obstacle.
- Think about weight-loss methods that you have used in the past. How many of the factors that predict successful weight loss and sustained weight loss were part of these methods? Are there things that you could have done differently to include more factors?
- What do you see as your "happy" weight and when do you see yourself achieving it? If your answer is a weight that is less than 90% of your current body weight and your time frame for reaching that weight is in less than six months, rethink your expectations. A reasonable goal is a loss of 10% of your current weight over six months. Start with that goal—you may very well surprise yourself by exceeding it!
- Identify at least three people you know who have successfully lost weight and are keeping it off. Find out about their experience—

what method they used, what strategies and approaches they took to make it work for them, and what they are doing to sustain the weight loss. Compare what they tell you about the factors of successful weight loss, the factors for sustained weight loss, and the basic components of a weight-loss program.

- Remind yourself often and with confidence that sustained weight loss is possible. Your body will not undermine your achievements by slowing metabolism so that you gain the weight back.

# Chapter 2

# Do those extra few pounds really matter?

A large number of us gain weight each year. In fact, adding pounds as we add years is so commonplace that we've come to accept it as a natural part of the aging process. We have also come to expect that we are likely to develop common health problems, like high blood pressure and diabetes. Consider for a moment, however, how these extra few pounds may be increasing your risk for developing these medical conditions. Read on to learn why a few extra pounds do matter, how you can halt the gain, and how losing a little pays back a lot.

# Myth 2 A few extra pounds don't matter

*Believers Beware!*

A few extra pounds hardly seem worth worrying about. Gaining a little is better than gaining a lot. Being a little overweight but not obese may be a cosmetic issue, but it is not a health issue.

Weight gain is just part of getting older. In fact, it is a natural part of the aging process. The body's metabolism slows over time, so it burns fewer calories. We're not as active as we were in our younger years. Who has the time or energy to play and run around the way we did when we were children?

As the body ages, it doesn't function as efficiently. It is very common for blood pressure to go up and for blood cholesterol to rise. People who are prone to getting diabetes have problems with high blood sugar. Cars often don't work as well when they get older. It's no surprise that the human body doesn't work as well either.

For most of us, fighting off weight gain is not worth the time or effort it takes. Given the health risks of yo-yo dieting, it is smarter to live with a few extra pounds than lose and gain over and over again.

## Kernels of Truth

There is a kernel of truth in the myth that a little extra weight is nothing to worry about. Within the relatively wide range of healthy weights, there is not a lot of evidence that some extra weight within that range is harmful to your health. However, once you leave that safe harbor of the healthy weight range, the negative health consequences begin to mount very quickly.

The myth of the weight gain–aging connection also has a kernel of truth. Several studies have found that Americans gain an average of 0.4 to 1.8 pounds each year during their adult lives.

**HOW WEIGHT GAIN ADDS UP: THE AVERAGE WEIGHT, BY DECADE, OF WOMEN AND MEN IN THE UNITED STATES**

| Age | Woman | Man |
|---|---|---|
| 20s | 132 pounds | 168 pounds |
| 30s | 144 pounds | 179 pounds |
| 40s | 149 pounds | 182 pounds |
| 50s | 158 pounds | 185 pounds |

*Source:* Adapted from data from NHANES III (1988–1994).

It is also true that body composition—that is the amount of muscle, fat, and other components that make up the body—changes as we get older. Some of this change results from age-related decreases in hormone levels. For example, a man's body gradually produces less testosterone, causing a reduction in muscle and an increase in body fat, especially around the abdomen. In women, estrogen drops in the years around menopause and causes a similar increase in fat around the waist.

## The Whole Truth

### BMI Demystified

Before getting into the whole truth, let's explain a term that will help you better understand weight and weight loss: Body Mass Index (BMI). BMI is the standard used around the world to determine whether a

# Personal Triumph

## Joe Harasym

FLORIDA

Joe Harasym put on weight slowly over the years but never took weight loss seriously. "Throughout my adult life, I was involved with crazy diets, like eating just grapefruit, drinking only weight-loss shakes, and even fasting for a few days. I was always trying something new, but I never really put my mind to it. I just accepted weight gain as a natural part of getting older.

*"I started Weight Watchers at 247 pounds and reached my first goal weight of 217."*

"Now that I am retired, my wife and I go on a lot of cruises. One day I was browsing through photographs that were taken on one of our cruises. I really didn't like what I saw in photos of myself and told my wife that it was time to do something about it. Two of our daughters-in-law were on Weight Watchers, so my wife and I both joined. I started Weight Watchers at 247 pounds and reached my first goal weight of 217. I lost even more weight, and now I maintain a weight of about 161 pounds. I know that I can lose any weight that I gain on a cruise or vacation."

Joe now knows that gaining weight does not have to be a part of the second spring of his life.

person's weight is healthy, overweight, or obese. For most people, BMI is strongly related to the amount of body fat you carry. You could calculate your BMI using your body weight, your height, and the BMI formula, but it is far easier to look up your BMI on a chart like the one below. To determine your BMI category, find your height in inches in the column on the left, run your finger across to the range that includes your current weight in pounds, then look up to the top of that column for your BMI range and category. This chart applies to both women and men.

**BODY MASS INDEX AND WEIGHT CLASSIFICATIONS**

| BMI | 19 or Lower | 19.0–24.9 | 25.0–29.9 | 30 or Higher |
|---|---|---|---|---|
| BMI Category | Underweight | Healthy | Overweight | Obese |
| Height (inches) | Body Weight (pounds) | | | |
| | Less than | | | More than |
| 58 | 90 | 91–118 | 119–142 | 143 |
| 59 | 93 | 94–123 | 124–147 | 148 |
| 60 | 96 | 97–127 | 128–152 | 153 |
| 61 | 99 | 100–131 | 132–157 | 158 |
| 62 | 103 | 104–135 | 136–163 | 164 |
| 63 | 106 | 107–140 | 141–168 | 169 |
| 64 | 109 | 110–144 | 145–173 | 174 |
| 65 | 113 | 114–149 | 150–179 | 180 |
| 66 | 117 | 118–154 | 155–185 | 186 |
| 67 | 120 | 121–158 | 159–190 | 191 |
| 68 | 124 | 125–163 | 164–197 | 197 |
| 69 | 127 | 128–168 | 169–202 | 203 |
| 70 | 131 | 132–173 | 174–208 | 209 |
| 71 | 135 | 136–178 | 179–214 | 215 |
| 72 | 139 | 140–183 | 184–220 | 221 |
| 73 | 143 | 144–188 | 189–226 | 227 |
| 74 | 147 | 148–193 | 194–232 | 233 |
| 75 | 151 | 152–199 | 200–239 | 240 |
| 76 | 155 | 156–204 | 205–245 | 246 |

*Source:* Adapted from http://www.nhlbi.nih.gov/guidelines/obesity/bmi_tbl.pdf.

*Have you ever heard . . .*

**"I am not overweight, I just have big bones."**

This statement has its roots in body weight tables that were used over twenty years ago. Before BMI became the standard, people compared their weight to an "ideal body weight" using height and weight tables that were developed by a major insurance company. These tables listed different weight ranges for people who had a "small," "medium," or "large" frame. Needless to say, the ideal body weight was not based on a scientific standard—it was based on the body weights of a group of people who had purchased life insurance from the insurance company. The company divided the range of body weights for each height into thirds and called the lowest third "small frame," the middle third "medium frame," and the highest third "large frame." Furthermore, the group was made up of primarily white men. The BMI offers a far more accurate evaluation of your body weight.

Dozens of scientific and medical organizations have agreed that a BMI between 19 and 24.9 is in the healthy range, a BMI between 25 and 29.9 is overweight, and a BMI of 30 or more is obese. These definitions are based on research showing that the risk of disease goes up when BMI is over 25, and the risk of death increases if BMI goes over 30.

Here are a couple of examples to help you better understand the chart. The average woman in the United States is 64 inches tall and is in the healthy range if she weighs between 110 and 144 pounds. She is overweight if she weighs between 145 and 173 pounds; if she weighs 174 pounds or more, she is considered obese. The average man in the United States is 70 inches tall. If he weighs between 132 and 173 pounds, he is in the healthy range. If he weighs between 174 and 208 pounds, he is overweight, and he is obese at 209 pounds or more.

## Why Metabolism Slows Down

Muscle determines how fast the body's engine runs and how many calories the body burns over the course of a day. Muscle falls into the "use it or lose it" category—if your muscles are not active, they will shrink. Since we tend to get less active as we get older, our muscles become smaller, and, as a result, our metabolism and calorie burning slow down. Research has shown that the impact of age-related changes in hormones is much smaller than the impact of muscle loss from lack of use.

Even if your weight stays the same as you get older, the amount of fat and muscle on your body will change. This is not the result of aging per se. Because adults become less active as they get older, they're likely to have more body fat and less lean tissue than in their younger years. A study published in *Nutrition* found a clear link between activity and body composition. People who were more physically active in their daily lives and through regular exercise had more muscle. The study also found that weight and body fat increased with age.

Any weight gain during adulthood is likely to be body fat because most adults are not active enough to build muscle. Some studies suggest that by age 55, the average person in the United States has added over 37 pounds of fat during his or her adult years!

Here's the good news. According to the American College of Sports Medicine, as part of a regular physical activity routine, muscle-building strength training can slow down muscle loss and help keep metabolism revved up.

## The Link between Weight and Health

Weight and health are strongly related to each other. Disease risk goes up slowly as weight gain pushes you out of the healthy weight range and into the overweight range. Your risk of disease and death increase significantly if extra weight puts you in the obese range. One study reported that obesity in middle age reduces life expectancy by seven years.

The list of weight-related diseases continues to grow. Increased weight raises blood lipids (cholesterol and triglycerides) and blood pressure, which are heart disease risk factors. Weight gain impairs the body's ability to handle glucose (blood sugar) and contributes to a pre-diabetic condition called insulin resistance. Other medical conditions that are associated with increased weight include certain cancers, osteoarthritis of the knees and other weight-bearing joints, gastrointestinal tract disturbances, interrupted sleep and sleep apnea, and reduced fertility. To date, obesity has been linked with more than thirty medical conditions.

As weight goes out of the healthy range, risk increases for

- Heart disease
- High blood pressure
- Stroke
- Diabetes
- Several forms of cancer
- Metabolic syndrome (Syndrome X)
- Gallbladder disease
- Gout

It is not just big gains that carry ill health effects—the consequences of gradual or modest weight gain add up quickly. Even 10 or 20 extra pounds increases the risk of death among adults, as shown in a large study published in the *New England Journal of Medicine*. A recently published study found that just a 5% increase in the BMI over time had a negative impact on simple body functions like walking. Research on women, weight gain, and cancer found that women who gained 21 to 30 pounds since age 18 and were not on hormone replacement therapy were 40% more likely to get breast cancer than women who had gained no more than 5 pounds. The risk increased as the women's weight increased. Similarly, another study found an 8% increase in the risk of postmenopausal breast cancer for every 11 pounds gained.

## Your Shape Matters

Is your body shaped more like an apple or a pear? When it comes to weight and health, being shaped like an apple carries greater health risks than being shaped like a pear.

You are apple-shaped if your body fat has settled around your belly. Men are genetically predisposed to gain weight around their belly, although there are exceptions. Having an apple-shaped body means that you have too much abdominal fat. Abdominal fat increases your risk of heart disease, diabetes, and breast cancer following menopause.

Pear-shaped bodies store more fat in the buttocks and hips. Women tend to gain weight on the hips and thighs. Whatever your shape, however, BMI is still important because it is linked with overall body fat. Chances are, if your BMI is high, your waist circumference will be high too.

### How to Evaluate Your Abdominal Fat

- Using a cloth measuring tape, like the one used by tailors, measure around the widest area between your belly button and the top of your hips.
- For men, if this measurement is more than 40 inches, you have abdominal obesity.
- For women, if this measurement is more than 35 inches, you have abdominal obesity.

## A Closer Look at Weight and Heart Disease

Heart disease is the leading killer of both men and women; 54% of all deaths result from heart disease. Being overweight or obese or having too much abdominal fat are strongly associated with heart disease risk factors including an increase in total and LDL ("bad") cholesterol, triglycerides, and blood pressure. Overweight, obesity, and abdominal fat increase the risk of diabetes, which is a heart disease risk factor.

# *Personal Triumph*

## Donna Carter

NORTH CAROLINA

Donna Carter, a medical transcriptionist, was slim until she had her second child. Then she underwent major surgery and couldn't walk or lift anything for two months. She had gained weight during pregnancy and during her two months of inactivity. In addition, she was prescribed a medication associated with weight gain.

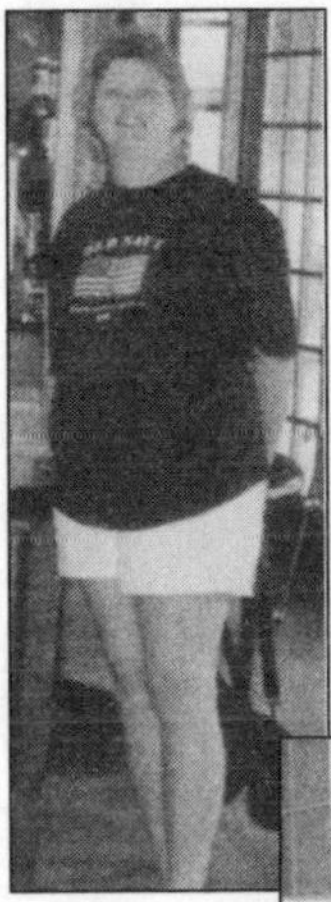

Donna's blood pressure had gone up as her weight did, so her doctor prescribed blood pressure medication and was considering prescribing a second medication. The defining moment for Donna to take control of her weight came when she was looking at some photographs.

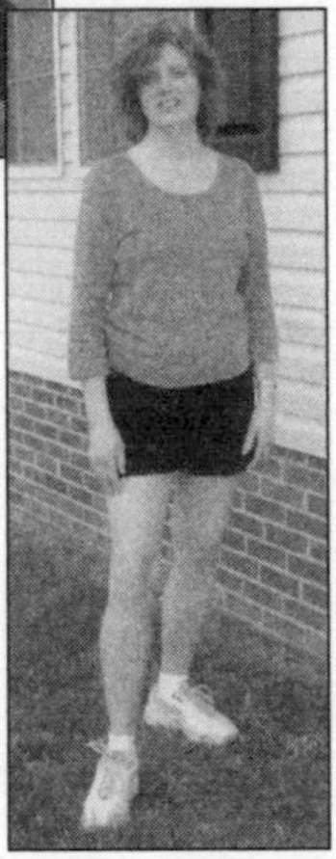

*"Weight Watchers is a healthier way to lose weight."*

"I saw a photo of myself that was taken at a pool. What a shock! I saw a skinny person every time I looked in the mirror, but the person in the photo was overweight. One of my coworkers is a Weight Watchers lifetime member, so I joined. Weight Watchers is a healthier way to lose weight."

Donna lost over 36 pounds to reach her goal weight and is able to control her blood pressure without any additional medication.

Being overweight also directly affects risk of heart disease—if your BMI is in the overweight range, your heart disease risk doubles compared to people with BMIs in the healthy weight range. If your BMI is in the obese category, your heart disease risk quadruples. Losing weight reduces the risk of heart disease.

## A Closer Look at Weight and Blood Cholesterol

Increased weight negatively affects cholesterol levels in the body, as well as some of the components of cholesterol. Your total cholesterol level is made up of three different types of cholesterol: LDL ("bad" cholesterol), VLDL (a mixture of triglycerides and cholesterol), and HDL ("good" cholesterol). Each type of cholesterol has a different function. For heart health, the goal is to decrease LDL cholesterol and increase HDL cholesterol, since LDL contributes to heart disease risk and HDL helps protect the heart. Increased weight creates problems by increasing LDL levels and decreasing HDL levels. It also drives up triglycerides, another type of fat in the blood. Weight loss improves the blood cholesterol and triglyceride levels.

**TARGET CHOLESTEROL LEVELS**

| | What It Stands For | Levels to Aim For (mg/dL) |
|---|---|---|
| TG | Triglyceride | Lower than 150 |
| LDL | Low-density lipoprotein | Lower than 100 is optimal; greater than 160 is high |
| HDL | High-density lipoprotein | Greater than 40 |

*Source:* Adapted from the American Heart Association (http://www.americanheart.org).

## A Closer Look at Weight and High Blood Pressure

If we could eliminate overweight and obesity in our country, we could eliminate between 40% and 70% of the medical diagnoses of high blood pressure. Societies where people don't gain much weight as they get older do not experience this increase in high blood pressure. The first thing a doctor tells an overweight or obese patient who has high blood pressure is to lose weight. Often this is enough to get his or her blood pressure under control even without any blood pressure medication.

## A Closer Look at Weight and Other Cardiovascular Problems

Increased weight is associated with increased risk of congestive heart failure, a frequent complication of obesity and a major cause of death. Obesity changes the heart size and structure, preventing it from working properly.

Obesity also dramatically increases the risk of ischemic stroke, which is like a heart attack that happens in the brain. Compared to a woman with a BMI in the healthy range, a woman with a BMI greater than 27 has a 75% higher risk of ischemic stroke, and a woman with a BMI greater than 32 has a 137% higher risk. Losing weight helps reduce the risk of both of these problems.

## A Closer Look at Weight and Diabetes

Perhaps the strongest association between weight gain, metabolic abnormalities, and disease risk is found with type 2 diabetes. (Type 1 diabetes typically affects younger people and is caused by the pancreas not producing insulin.) A majority of people who have type 2 diabetes are also overweight, and the incidence of type 2 diabetes is increasing as the population becomes more overweight.

About 90% of people with diabetes have type 2 diabetes, which develops when the insulin-producing pancreas cannot keep up with the body's need for insulin, a hormone that helps blood sugar enter cells. With weight gain, cells in the body do not respond properly to insulin, causing an unhealthy rise in blood sugar levels. This is known as insulin resistance. The pancreas produces insulin, but the insulin no longer works effectively.

Weight gain dramatically increases diabetes risk. The risk goes up with weight increases after age 18. The risk also increases about 25% for every unit increase in BMI over 22. One study estimated that more than one-quarter of new cases of type 2 diabetes could be attributed to a weight gain of 11 pounds or more.

If we eliminate adult weight gain and obesity, we could eliminate over 80% of all type 2 diabetes. It is not surprising that one of the first treatment recommendations for type 2 diabetes is to lose weight.

## A Closer Look at Weight and the Metabolic Syndrome

Many people have never even heard of the metabolic syndrome, also known as Syndrome X. Until recently, most physicians had never heard of the metabolic syndrome either. Yet this condition—a combination of blood lipid abnormalities, high blood pressure, and elevated blood sugar—affects almost one-quarter of the adult population in the United States. The major underlying cause of the metabolic syndrome is obesity, in particular, increased abdominal fat.

Five different conditions make up the metabolic syndrome:

1. High blood triglycerides
2. Low HDL cholesterol
3. High blood pressure
4. Elevated blood sugar
5. Increased waist circumference (as mentioned earlier in this chapter, greater than 40 inches in men and greater than 35 inches in women)

The metabolic syndrome is rapidly becoming a significant medical problem because it increases so many risk factors for heart disease and diabetes. Weight loss is the only effective treatment for this condition.

## A Closer Look at Weight and Cancer

Recent studies from the National Cancer Institute and other research institutions suggest that over 20% of all cancer is related to overweight or obesity. For years, researchers have commented that certain forms of cancer with a link to hormones (for example, breast and endometrial cancer in women, prostate cancer in men) are associated with weight gain, overweight, and obesity. As summarized in a government report on overweight and obesity, obesity increases the risk of breast cancer after menopause because body fat produces the hormone estrogen. Even weight gain not to the point of obesity can be a problem: gaining more than 20 pounds between age 18 and midlife doubles a woman's breast cancer risk. The risk of colon cancer and other gastrointestinal tract cancers that do not appear to have a connection to hormones also goes up as one's weight increases.

### Weight Loss Improves Your Health

So it is clear that gaining even a little bit of weight is not good for a person's health. Thankfully, the same cannot be said for the reverse—

*Have you ever heard…*

**"If getting thinner is good, getting very thin must be even better."**

The best goal is to reduce weight into the healthy weight range, which is quite broad and typically spans at least 20 to 40 pounds. For most health benefits, there is no real evidence that losing so much that you are near the bottom of the healthy weight range is any better than being near the top of the healthy weight range.

For example, Jim is 5'9" tall and weighs 155 pounds, for a BMI of 23. According to the healthy weight range for his height, he could lose 27 pounds, lowering his weight to 128, which would give him a BMI of 19. It is best to find a comfortable and sustainable weight within the healthy weight range, if possible.

Keep in mind, though, that even if you can't get into the healthy weight range, losing smaller amounts of weight can carry significant health benefits.

# *Personal Triumph*

## Ron Dieckman

ILLINOIS

At 6'6" and 280 pounds, Ron Dieckman didn't consider himself overweight. "I was slim in my youth and always wished that I was bigger. So as an adult, I liked being big. I looked like a middle linebacker, with all my weight around my midsection. I never considered myself to be overweight.

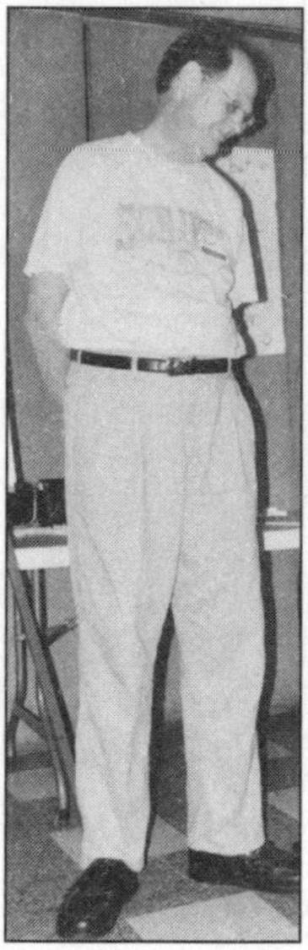

"When my wife, Sherri, attended her first Weight Watchers meeting, I went along to encourage her. She went to register, and I sat in the meeting room saving her a chair. She came into the room and told me that she signed both of us up. I looked at her and said, 'Us? I don't need this. Are you telling me I'm overweight?' Now I know that I used to be overweight. I also know that I'm not overweight anymore."

*"Now I know that I used to be overweight. I also know that I'm not overweight anymore."*

Ron lost over 50 pounds to reach his goal weight. Since then, Ron has joined the Weight Watchers staff and is helping others to learn when they are overweight and how to take the extra weight off.

losing a little weight is very good. It takes only a small weight loss—as little as 5%—to gain health benefits. For a person who weighs 200 pounds, that's just 10 pounds!

Weight loss is vital in the treatment and prevention of heart disease, unhealthy blood cholesterol levels, heart failure, high blood pressure, type 2 diabetes, and other chronic diseases. A loss of just 5% of body weight can reduce, eliminate, or prevent these conditions in many overweight people. The news is even better if you sustain your weight loss. Maintaining a loss of 10% of your original body weight improves the body's response to insulin, aids blood sugar control, controls or prevents high blood pressure, and improves triglyceride, HDL cholesterol, and LDL cholesterol levels. The health benefits are especially profound when you lose excess abdominal fat.

Here is a summary of just a few of the benefits of losing a modest amount of weight, defined as weight loss of 5% to 10% of initial body weight:

- Reduce risk of breast cancer, in particular, if the weight is lost before age 45.
- Drop blood pressure (both the upper and lower numbers) by 10 points for every 20 pounds of weight lost.
- Increase HDL cholesterol incrementally for every BMI change downward of one unit—for example, from 29 to 28.
- Reduce incidence of diabetes by 58%.

The link between weight loss and diabetes prevention is particularly compelling. In the Diabetes Prevention Program, a lifestyle program that was conducted at several research institutions and included weight loss and physical activity components, participants dramatically reduced their risk of developing diabetes with a weight loss of just 7%. The results of this lifestyle program were similar to those observed in people on medication.

## The Bottom Line

Even being a little overweight is not a good idea. Specifically, weight gain that pushes your weight out of the healthy BMI weight range begins to increase your disease risk. Finding a comfortable weight within the healthy range for your height—a weight corresponding to a BMI between 19 and 24.9—is best.

Our message to you is very clear: *Try to achieve and sustain a goal weight that is in the healthy weight range.* Once your weight creeps into the overweight range, the myth that a little extra weight is nothing to worry about can be very hazardous to your health.

Raise a yellow caution flag in your mind if your bathroom scale is consistently telling you that you are 5 or more pounds heavier than you were in the past. Unfortunately, the relationship between even a small amount of weight gain and adverse health consequences is quite strong.

There is solid evidence that even a relatively small amount of weight loss can improve your health significantly. Losing 5% to 10% of your starting weight lowers disease risk. If you've lost weight before but gained it back, you may be concerned about even trying to lose. Don't let that prevent you from losing weight again—you can learn how to sustain your weight loss and avoid the loss-gain cycle. You *can* stop the weight gain and sustain a lower weight that will benefit your health!

## *Personal Triumph*

**Joe Harasym**
FLORIDA

Joe Harasym, whom you met earlier in this chapter, had been under a doctor's treatment for over twenty years for high cholesterol and high blood pressure and was on medications for both conditions. His health improved dramatically after he became a Weight Watchers member.

"I never put my mind to anything like I did Weight Watchers. Joining with my wife was a big help because we eat the same foods, and that makes things easier. As I lost weight and ate more sensibly by cutting out fats and fried stuff, my cholesterol dropped down to 126 from 240, and my doctor cut my cholesterol medication dosage in half. My blood pressure had been high for the past thirty years. Now it's normal, at 120/80."

> *"I never put my mind to anything like I did Weight Watchers."*

Joe now looks forward to his annual physical.

# Action Steps

If you have gained weight as an adult, you are not alone. There is no way that any of us can turn back the hands of time. That does not mean, however, that the extra pounds should be accepted as part of the aging process. Every year you carry the extra weight means a higher risk of developing several diseases. Losing the weight will bring those risks down. Now is the time to do a weight and health check to find out where you are so that you can make decisions about where you want to go.

- Think back to your 18th birthday. Do you weigh the same now as you did then? If you have gained weight, how many pounds have you gained?
- Determine if you are at a healthy weight, overweight, or obese by finding your BMI.
- Take your waist circumference. Is it over the recommended measurement?
- If you have not done so in the past year, schedule yourself for a complete physical. Ask you doctor what impact, if any, your weight has on your current health status. Find out and make a record of your blood lipid levels, blood pressure, and fasting blood sugar.
- Set a realistic weight goal.
  - If you are at a healthy weight and have not gained weight as an adult, a realistic goal is to prevent weight gain.
  - If you are currently gaining weight, a reasonable first goal is to hold your weight steady to stop the gain.
  - If you are ready to lose weight, aim to lose 5% to 10% of your initial weight. Once that is achieved and celebrated, set another goal or a series of realistic goals until you reach your ultimate goal weight (a weight within the healthy BMI range).
- Choose a weight-loss method and approach (more on this later) that leads to sustained weight loss.

# Chapter 3

# Is willpower the key to weight loss?

It would be wonderful if losing weight were simply a matter of willpower. In fact, willpower is often cited as the only true factor for weight-loss success. The reality is that willpower is just one part of the weight-loss equation and its role is often overrated. Read on to learn how to harness the willpower that lies within each of us and combine it with other important factors so that you can achieve lasting weight loss.

# Myth 3 Willpower is the key to successful weight loss

*Believers Beware!*

Losing weight is not really all that complicated. All it takes is eating less and exercising more. If people cannot do these two simple things, it can only be due to one of two reasons. The first reason is a lack of knowledge. After all, a lot of people do not know enough about food and activity, and how they influence weight loss. The good news is that this reason can be easily fixed with education. Then all they have to do put that knowledge into action and they will lose weight.

If they have been educated and do not lose weight, there is only one reason: lack of willpower. Willpower is an inborn mental trait—either you have it or you don't. It is not something that you can learn, buy, or teach yourself. If you do not have willpower, you cannot lose weight.

## Kernels of Truth

The mental aspects of weight loss are critically important. Without mental strategies for making wise food choices, dealing with stress, making physical activity a priority, and dozens of other actions, weight loss is virtually impossible.

Successful weight management—losing weight and keeping it off—requires a commitment. Some people call this commitment willpower. You have to commit to making smart choices and sticking to your choices for weight loss to be successful.

Knowledge is power. The more you know about food, physical activity, and the path to sustainable weight loss, the greater your ability to make smart choices. Knowing which foods are satisfying for you and also happen to be lower in calories makes weight loss attainable. Likewise, knowing how to exercise in a way that helps your body build muscle, burns a lot of calories, and is enjoyable can boost your weight-loss efforts. You can't lose weight without knowing what to do.

*Have you ever heard . . .*

**"People who are overweight just don't have willpower."**

Willpower is a part of weight loss, but to believe that people who are overweight simply lack willpower is simply wrong. Losing weight and sustaining weight loss require much more than willpower. They require a comprehensive weight-loss method that includes having a positive mindset, paying attention to food choices, regular physical activity, and creating a supportive atmosphere.

# *Personal Triumph*

## Rebecca Hill

CALIFORNIA

Rebecca Hill was slim when she started working as a postproduction coordinator on the first *American Idol* show. Work-related stress caused her to change her eating habits and eat virtually nonstop. Rebecca gained between 30 and 40 pounds and was heading higher.

*"I need structure to help me stay focused, which is why Weight Watchers works so well for me."*

"My weight issues reached a turning point after I ate two whole boxes of cookies in the time that it took my husband to do some banking at an ATM. I decided to join Weight Watchers because my mother had been on Weight Watchers for years and made it a part of her life.

"I have the least willpower of anyone I know. I need structure to help me stay focused, which is why Weight Watchers works so well for me. Because of the plan that I am on, I have concrete structure that helps me make my wise food choices every day. At the same time, I enjoy the flexibility that Weight Watchers provides. I can eat anything and everything, which I still do!

"Self-monitoring also is key for me. I'm an emotional eater, so I have to take life meal by meal and day by day to stay on top of my eating. If I didn't monitor my eating, I would be lost at sea."

Rebecca reached her goal weight by losing over 41 pounds.

## The Whole Truth

### Willpower Is Only One Part of the Answer

Believing that weight loss and weight maintenance are simply a matter of willpower can be dangerous. Yet it's a very common conviction. When describing their history of weight loss, many people talk about the vast amounts of energy spent on exerting willpower. If weight loss does not occur—or more commonly, the weight that is lost snaps back—blame is put on a lack of willpower. This pattern is self-defeating. Getting over the hurdle of believing only in willpower and into the process of establishing a comprehensive weight-loss method is the answer.

### Knowledge Isn't Everything, Either

Knowledge is about more than numbers. Knowing how many calories are in a cookie does not tell you whether to or how to include that cookie in your eating plan. Knowing how many calories you burn in an aerobics class does not tell you whether that amount of physical activity will help you lose weight. Successful weight loss requires understanding the big picture, not just knowing pieces of information.

However, knowing about weight management behaviors, making wise choices, eating healthfully, enjoying food, and doing physical activities that you enjoy can be a powerful set of tools for taking control of your weight for good.

### Learn Flexible Restraint

Let's define one aspect of willpower as the ability to hold yourself back from eating or overeating when you're around food. Weight-loss scientists call this *dietary restraint*. It describes how tightly a person regulates her or his food intake. For example, highly restrained dieters are very precise about how much they eat, say, 200 calories for breakfast, 300 calories for lunch, 700 calories for dinner, and no snacks. You probably know people who add up the calories in every bite, read every label, and talk a lot about how they watch what they're eating. These are highly restrained eaters. Do you often wish that you could be more of a restrained eater?

*You may be surprised to learn that a very high level of dietary restraint is associated with obesity, not with successful weight management, and is also linked to a lack of success in weight-loss attempts.*

> How can high levels of dietary restraint be connected with excess weight? While the specifics are an intense area of scientific investigation, the simple answer is that high restraint levels cannot be sustained for extended periods of time. Invariably, the restraint is abandoned and overeating occurs. People who tend to have high levels of dietary restraint are also prone to on again, off again weight-loss practices.

The flip side of dietary restraint is *dietary disinhibition*—lack of inhibition when eating. We have all opened a bag of cookies, eaten a couple, then thought, since I started them, I may as well finish them. Interestingly, although disinhibition is the opposite of restraint, high levels of dietary disinhibition are also associated with obesity and lack of weight-loss success.

So here is the quandary: If dietary restraint is linked with overweight and unsuccessful weight loss and dietary disinhibition is also linked with extra pounds, what should you do? *The answer is to find the middle ground with a strategy called flexible restraint.*

Flexible restraint means moderately controlling your eating. After all, eating as much of any food as you want and doing so whenever you feel like it is not going to help you with weight loss. Your eating plan needs enough structure to give you the security and comfort that you are in control of your eating. But the plan also needs enough flexibility so that you won't feel trapped, deprived, or restricted by overly strict rules. The key is to find a balance you can maintain.

If you have recently gone out to dinner, gotten together with friends, or attended a gathering where food was served, you know that there are times when a little overeating is inevitable. A strategy of flexible restraint allows for slight overeating one day followed by eating a bit less the next meal or the next day and/or increasing physical activity to make up for the overeating.

Flexible restraint allows you to adapt to the ups and downs of daily life. No more of the I'm on my diet/I'm off my diet mentality that is a common weight-loss downfall. An eating style that incorporates flexible restraint takes away the pressure of needing superhuman amounts of willpower for dietary restraint. It also helps avoid the total loss of willpower associated with dietary disinhibition.

Sound too good to be true? Not only does flexible restraint work but it also appears to be connected to long-term weight management.

Researchers measure levels of dietary restraint and disinhibition with detailed tests. To find out if you are a restrained or a disinhibited eater, have an honest chat with yourself about how you regulate your eating. The questions below can help you get started.

There are several ways to look at or define eating flexibility and structure, and the same approach does not work for everyone. Chapter 9 can help you learn how to balance flexibility, freedom, and structure to best fit your lifestyle.

**Are you more of a restrained eater?**

- Do you count every calorie, ounce, or half a ***POINTS*** value*?
- Do you try to have perfect control over your eating?
- Do you feel stressed in situations with a lot of food choices?

*The ***POINTS***® Food System, a proprietary component of the Weight Watchers program, is explained in the Afterword.

**Are you more of a disinhibited eater?**

- Is it hard for you to stop eating?
- Do you finish the whole box or bag rather than taking a reasonable portion?
- Does overeating at one meal lead to more overeating at the next meal?

# Personal Triumph

## Christine Bogosian

CALIFORNIA

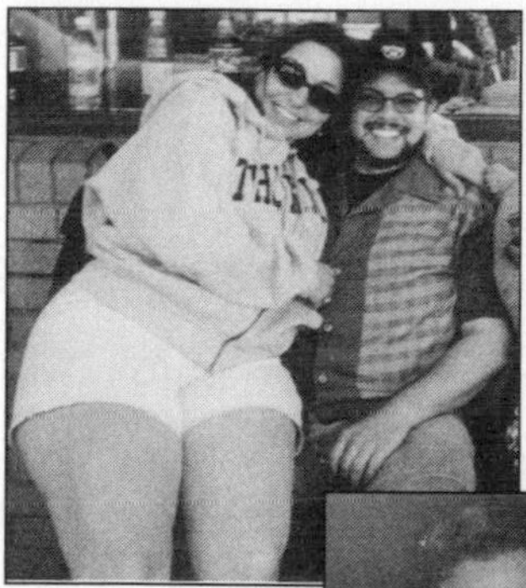

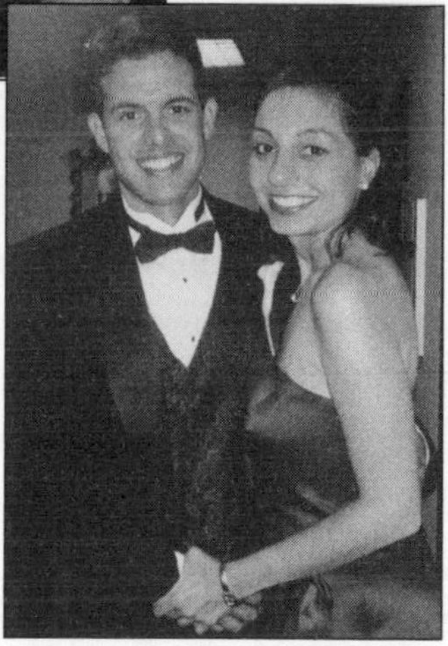

Christine Bogosian is an attorney. A former competitive ice skater, Christine gained weight during law school.

"I was not paying attention to what and how much I was eating. I tried to be more aware and to make better food choices, but it was too much work for me. I just gave up. I also had little time for physical activity.

"Once I joined Weight Watchers, I learned to make time for activity. I also really enjoy my food. I am a true believer in not depriving myself. If I want a piece of chocolate, I first ask myself if it is really worth it. If the answer is yes, then I let myself have a little piece. I know that if I deprive myself, I will end up eating the whole box."

*"Once I joined Weight Watchers, I learned to make time for activity."*

Approximately nine months after joining Weight Watchers, Christine reached her goal weight by losing 56 pounds.

## Willpower Versus Want Power

Managing your weight means finding the balance between willpower and *want power*. Earlier in this chapter, willpower was defined as the mental strength to set limits for yourself. Want power is your desire and motivation—the forces that drive you to behave in a certain way. Want power is not just about food; it is about your entire weight management strategy.

Motivation changes over time. A single spark—losing weight for your wedding, a hurtful comment by a friend or coworker, a lecture from your doctor—may motivate you to lose weight. In fact, most successful dieters can pinpoint the spark that marked the start of their weight-loss journey. Sometimes the sparks are positive; sometimes they are negative. What they have in common is they are strong enough to motivate taking the first step on the weight-loss path. Don't be surprised if you feel ambivalent during the course of your weight-loss journey—there will be times when you are fully committed and times when you are not so sure.

Before you select a weight management program, have a talk with yourself about what you want (want power) and don't want (will power). Select a program that will help you be successful by satisfying your wants (within reason, of course) without requiring superhuman amounts of willpower. In your mind, see and feel the changes that weight loss will bring. And don't expect to be perfect—nobody is that strong.

*Have you ever heard . . .*

**"Losing weight is just a matter of getting real with yourself."**

While it is important to face the realities in your life, you also have to find approaches for dealing with an environment that is filled with food temptations and reasons to avoid physical activity.

## Motivations Change

Here is a really surprising research finding: how motivated people are at the beginning of weight loss has nothing to do with whether their weight loss will be successful. We all know people who are gung ho when they decide to lose weight. And then we are shocked when they do not achieve lasting results. What happened?

There is a difference between short-term and long-term motivation. Short-term motivation is what motivates you right now. Long-term motivation is the bigger picture. If you turn back to chapter 1 and look at the list of factors linked with sustainable weight loss, you'll see that motivation is not on the list. Health improvements and positive coping skills, however, are. A person can be motivated long term by the prospect of better health or by being able to deal with food in a healthier way.

It is hard to develop long-term motivation and turn it into daily strategies that fit within the fabric of your life. It may help to come up with several short-term motivations that have immediate feedback to keep you going as well as strategies to feed those motivations. Include sustaining weight loss in your thoughts as well as the weight loss that you are working on at the moment.

**SHORT-TERM MOTIVATORS AND STRATEGIES**

| When | Motivator | Strategy |
|---|---|---|
| First few weeks | Quick, noticeable weight loss | Focus just on food; master the eating plan |
| Weight loss hits plateau | Look and feel better already | Talk to others who have gotten stuck; share ideas |
| Goal weight reached | Compliments from others | Monitor weight closely; keep exercising |
| Maintain goal weight short term | Knowing that you have done it | Celebrate and reward self; write down the benefits you are feeling |
| Maintain goal weight long term | Better health; feel better; more energy | Strengthen coping skills; enjoy life |

# *Personal Triumph*

## Michelle Krischke

TEXAS

*"Through Weight Watchers, I learned the most amazing thing about willpower."*

Michelle Krischke, a credit assistant, tried every diet out there in her lifelong struggle with her weight. She remembers her mother making her clothes, buying clothing patterns for chubby children since she couldn't fit into regular-size clothing. Michelle tried everything—exercise, medications, low-carbohydrate diets, injections, and diet pills.

"They all worked, but the problem was that I never learned how to eat and how to manage food temptations. Whenever I reached my goal, I went back to my old ways and gained the weight back. Then I joined Weight Watchers.

"Through Weight Watchers, I learned the most amazing thing about willpower. My cravings go away when I'm eating properly, and that gives me willpower. I have found alternatives to food temptations that trigger my eating, like lower-calorie ice cream pops instead of regular ice cream, and soy chips instead of potato chips. Those alternatives really fulfill my needs."

Michelle lost 49 pounds to reach her goal weight.

### Food Temptations Differ

Which foods are hard for you to resist? Do you feel weak in the knees when you smell french fries? Or do the chocolate bars at the checkout counter call your name? New research studying the effects of food on the brain is finding that different people respond differently to the smell, appearance, and taste of food.

The amount of willpower it takes to say no to a food is directly linked to how tempting that food is to *you*. Your brain is wired differently from your friend's, so you will need to work harder to avoid or limit french fries. You may even decide to avoid fast-food outlets and other places that smell like fries, especially when you're hungry or feeling less strong.

Coming to terms with your food temptations does not mean that you should give up because biology is making you fat! Once you understand your unique temptations, you can deal with and develop strategies to overcome them.

## Mind and Body Working Together

Successful weight loss means getting your mind and your body to work together as one team. The mind can be a powerful ally if you learn to listen to your mental cues about eating and other weight-related issues and develop sound approaches to deal with these issues. But the body, especially the stomach, often seems to have a mind of its own!

Mind–body balance is not about the mind imposing tight restrictions on the body, like not eating after 8:00 P.M. or severely restricting calories. It is about finding a livable eating structure and lifestyle that keeps the mind *and* the body happy.

Here's an example of what can go wrong with an out-of-balance strategy. The mind decides that skipping breakfast would be a good way to lose weight. However, skipping breakfast restricts calories right at the point when the body needs them the most to face the challenges of the day. People who skip breakfast tend to make up for the missing breakfast calories, and more, later in the day because the body gets too hungry and overrides the mind—it needs food. Out-of-balance strategies can cause disinhibited eating, going for the whole box rather than one cookie. Tempting foods become even more tempting. It is not fair to blame this situation on a lack of willpower and self-discipline, but many people do.

It does not have to be that way. The mind can be a very powerful ally in a comprehensive program to effectively lose weight and keep it off. Learning, developing, and practicing coping skills improves your chances of weight-loss success.

## Talk the Talk, Walk the Walk

It is important to recognize that while mental strategies are necessary, they are not enough. Thoughts are useful only if they can change behavior. Talking the talk means walking the walk! You need to frame the mental strategy correctly.

Research by James Prochaska, a scientist who is famous for his studies on how people make changes, found that behavior techniques that help people cope with food-related situations increase the chance of successful weight loss. The key is to learn about approaches that other people have followed and discover the ones that work for you.

Developing new skills and habits takes time and effort. But participants from both the Weight Watchers Lifetime Member (LTM) Database and the National Weight Control Registry (NWCR) say that the amount of effort needed to sustain weight loss gets easier over time and that the effort is definitely worth it.

## Strategies Support Willpower

Chapter 1 introduced the basic components of a comprehensive weight-loss method: making positive changes, making wise food choices, being physically active, and living in a supportive environment. Let's look at how each of these can make it easier to use willpower for weight management.

Making positive changes includes developing and practicing techniques that reinforce your belief that you can lose weight and keep it off. Given the right tools, you can trust your ability to make smart choices that will help you reach your goals.

**Positive Changes Support Willpower**

- Visualize yourself at your goal weight.
- Rehearse food and activity strategies.
- Give yourself positive feedback.
- Remind yourself that you are making long-term lifestyle changes; you are not on a diet.

Making wise food choices is so important in our food-filled environment. We live in a world with an abundance of food that tastes good and is high in calories. You need a good knowledge of foods and food choices so that you can make smart decisions. You also need a healthy eating plan that you can follow every day but that allows enough flexibility for special events and changes in your routine. It also is important to support your willpower and do the little things that make it easier to stay the course.

**Food Choices Support Willpower**

- Avoid places that are filled with your food temptations, especially when you are hungry.
- Think ahead so that you have food that you want to eat when you want to eat it.
- Don't keep irresistible foods close at hand.
- Rehearse strategies to ask for what you want when you're away from home.

# Personal Triumph

**Rebecca Hill**
CALIFORNIA

Let's visit Rebecca Hill again, who admits that she does not get nearly enough physical activity. One of her goals is to get into a steady exercise routine.

"I exercise sporadically, just walking instead of driving down to the post office or walking to and from buildings at work. I know that exercise needs to be a part of my daily life if I want to achieve the health and fitness goals I have in mind for myself. I have the least willpower of anyone I know.

*"I believe that with the support of my Meeting Leader and fellow Weight Watchers members I will start an exercise program."*

"I told my Weight Watchers Meeting Leader and fellow members that I can't seem to get motivated and asked how I should start. Because having a lot of structure works so well for me when it comes to food, I got lots of ideas that would translate that approach into exercise. One suggestion was to sign up for a physical education class at my local college so that I have structure and accountability when it comes to exercise. Another was to schedule my exercise time into my date book and honor it as if it was a work meeting or getting together with a friend for dinner.

"I believe that with the support of my Meeting Leader and fellow Weight Watchers members I will start an exercise program."

Both Weight Watchers LTM Database and NWCR participants say that regular physical activity is an extremely important aspect of their weight-loss success. For weight management, heart health, and overall well-being, getting regular physical activity is one of the best choices you can make daily. Study after study has shown that regular physical activity is a key component of a comprehensive plan for sustainable weight loss. The obvious benefit is that physical activity burns calories and helps improve muscle tone. It makes you feel better, and it's easier to have willpower when you feel good. Physical activity reduces stress, which helps you focus on making smart decisions. Of course, physical activity alone is not enough.

**Physical Activity Supports Willpower**

- Schedule physical activity into your daily calendar.
- Keep exercise clothing in your car so that it's always handy.
- Join a class with an inspiring instructor.
- Choose activities that best fit your schedule and lifestyle.

We are programmed to want and need the company of others. Eating is one of our most social activities. Yet many people feel that when it comes to weight loss, they need to do it alone. (Chapter 10 further explores the role of people around you in managing your weight and the impact you have on them.) Assistance and encouragement from family and friends can be a tremendous boost to willpower. Being able to talk with people who are also striving to achieve a healthy body weight can be incredibly helpful. Getting insights and encouragement from those who are now maintaining weight loss is invaluable. In chapter 1, we listed the predictors of weight-loss success. Attendance in a weight-loss program was one of those predictors. The supportive atmosphere that is part of the program is no doubt a big contributor to weight-loss success.

**Creating a Supportive Atmosphere to Boost Your Willpower**

- Tell family and friends that you are trying to lose weight and ask for their support and understanding
- Share your success stories and bumps in the road with others
- Seek out people who have a positive outlook and avoid those who may try to sabotage you
- Attend a weight-loss program

## Strategies Need Plans

Would you set out on an unfamiliar destination without a road map or directions? Probably not. Likewise, achieving sustainable weight loss requires a map—a specific plan. While adopting a long-term mindset is very important, it is also important to break down the process by writing guidelines for yourself. Some people use a date book, others prefer electronic organizers, and many just use a piece of paper or an index card. You can include everything you're doing for the day: regularly scheduled appointments, appointments with doctors and dentists, and activities related to weight management such as exercise sessions and weekly meetings. Creating a schedule and following it helps you rely less on willpower to get through the day.

When it comes to food, it is important to have a daily plan that fits into your life as well as an overall plan that includes strategies for shopping and preparing food. You might schedule a weekly or twice-weekly shopping trip to a market that you know stocks high-quality fruits and vegetables, since fruits and vegetables are an important component of healthful eating and of eating for weight loss. Another option is to schedule an afternoon or evening for preparing and freezing foods so that you have healthy choices when you return home at the end of a long day. Keep fruits and vegetables on hand so that you

# *Personal Triumph*

**Michelle Krischke**
TEXAS

Michelle Krischke, whose story we told earlier in this chapter, feels that she learned a lot about herself by attending her Weight Watchers meeting each week.

"At my meetings I listened carefully to the information and discussion that took place. I was amazed how much everyone had in common. Every week, I came away with something—a way to handle a challenging situation, a tip to make my meals more interesting, or words of encouragement that boosted my motivation to succeed."

*"I was amazed how much everyone had in common."*

can grab a healthful snack without much thought. An attractive display in a fruit bowl in your kitchen increases the likelihood that you will grab a piece of fruit for a snack rather than high-calorie cookies or chocolates. Little steps like these take the pressure off willpower.

## The Bottom Line

Mental strategies matter. They are a vital part of a comprehensive weight-loss method. Use the power of mental strategies to your advantage. Make a long-term commitment to manage your weight, adopt a long-term mindset, think ahead, and establish proper structure and flexibility. By doing so, you can turn your mind into a healer . . . and your number one ally.

The more you know, the more likely you are to do the right thing. Knowledge about losing weight goes far deeper than knowing what to eat or how to exercise. It's a complex issue that has both mental and physical factors. Both need to be understood in order to be dealt with and mastered. You may not be able to learn how to have more willpower, but you can learn skills and techniques that make following a weight-loss program less stressful. You can also learn to harness the willpower you didn't know you had and gain strength from the people around you.

## Weight Loss That Lasts

# Action Steps

Successful weight loss is not simply a matter of exerting mind over matter. It requires knowing who you are, what you want, and having specific goals and strategies about how you are going to get there. The following steps will help you translate what you want into the will to make it happen:

- Evaluate your current eating habits as they relate to dietary restraint and dietary inhibition. What are your strengths and weaknesses?
- Choose a weight-loss method with a food component that supports the concept of flexible restraint. Extreme diets or diets that lend themselves to on-again, off-again eating can lead to dietary disinhibition and uncontrolled eating.
- Define what you want for yourself in terms of weight management. Evaluate the methods you are considering in relation to their ability to give you what you really want.
- Create a set of short- and longer-term goals. Determine what will motivate you to get from one goal to the next. Develop and implement strategies that will feed the motivators and help make them a reality.
- For each of the basic components of a comprehensive weight-loss method, think of at least four strategies you can implement today. Now implement them for a few days and see if they work for you. If they do, keep them. If they don't work for you, develop and test new strategies.
- Identify five of your temptation foods. Develop specific strategies for dealing with them in a way that will reinforce learning the skill of flexible restraint.

# Chapter 4

# Should I focus mostly on exercise?

Nobody is going to tell you that exercise is not a good thing. It offers many health benefits—better sleep, reduced stress, improved strength and muscle tone, and it puts you in a better mood. It also burns calories. So it makes sense that increasing physical activity be part of the weight-loss formula. But exercise as a weight-loss method has limitations. This chapter explores the effectiveness of exercise and its role in weight loss and maintenance.

# Myth 4 You can lose weight with exercise alone

*Believers Beware!*

Most diets fail because they focus on the wrong thing. Successful weight loss is not really about food; it is about exercise. The main focus of a weight-loss effort should be exercise because it will make the pounds come off faster and the loss will be maintained.

With all the technological changes in our daily lives, most of us are not getting enough exercise. People, especially guys, start gaining weight in their late 20s, then continue to gain weight into their 30s and 40s as work and family take up more of their time. With less time to exercise and be active, of course they gain weight. So it makes sense that getting back into exercise will melt away the pounds.

The commitment to exercise is not very demanding. Getting to the gym just a few times a week will make a huge difference in weight loss. And the more time spent at the gym, the faster the pounds will come off. It should take only a couple of hours a week for the next two or three months to lose the weight that has accumulated over the past ten or so years.

Going to the gym tones the body, flattens the stomach, and firms the thighs. It changes the shape of the body. Losing weight through dieting can't do that. So even if the pounds on the scale stay the same, that is okay; it just means that the fat is turning into muscle.

## Kernels of Truth

Numerous kernels of truth support the myth regarding exercise and weight loss. Let's start with the most obvious one: the average North American does not get enough exercise. We are all daily users of a variety of work-saving devices, like garage door openers, television remote controls, cordless telephones, and riding lawn mowers. A study done in Australia showed that we would need to walk 10 miles a day to make up for the decrease in the number of calories burned by daily activities since the 1800s.

Most people do not spend their free time being physically active. In 1997, less than one-third of adults in the United States got the recommended amount of physical activity and 40% of adults engaged in virtually no leisure-time physical activity.

Lack of exercise contributes to weight gain. Weight goes up when more calories are consumed than spent through activity.

**How the Body Spends Calories**

- Metabolism to keep the body functioning
- Physical activity
- Digesting and absorbing food

Beyond its role in weight control, exercise improves overall health. According to the Surgeon General's Report on Physical Activity and Health, benefits of regular physical activity include a lower risk of

- Heart disease
- High blood pressure or high cholesterol
- Premature death
- Colon and breast cancer
- Diabetes

Exercise has numerous other benefits beyond protection from diseases. It improves the health of muscles, bones, and joints. People who exercise perform better at recreational activities and even at work. Regular exercise also reduces stress and improves mental well-being. Depression and anxiety are less likely to occur in people who exercise regularly.

Losing fat and building muscle will help tone the body and put you into a smaller clothing size because a pound of muscle takes up a lot less space than a pound of fat. Picture a 1-pound package of lean meat or chicken from the grocery store; now picture four sticks of butter. They each weigh 1 pound, but the butter takes up more space than the meat.

*Have you ever heard . . .*

**"I am not overweight, I am muscular."**

A lot of people feel that measures of weight and overweight don't take muscle into account. It is true that body mass index (BMI) tables for height and weight misclassify some high-level athletes, like football players or body builders, as overweight when in fact they are very muscular. However, this applies to only a small number of athletes. For most of us, an overweight classification on the BMI table means that we are overweight from too much body fat.

# The Whole Truth

## Weight Gain Is Also Due to Overeating

While reduced physical activity is a significant contributor to weight gain, we are also eating more. The average American adult eats about 300 more calories per day than in 1970. In studies that have looked at where those calories are coming from, mixed grain dishes like pizza and tacos and calorie-containing beverages except milk top the list. Experts agree—the combination of eating more and moving less is behind the weight gain of the past thirty years.

Weight loss and weight gain are explained by the balance between

# Personal Triumph

## Sara Levitt

CALIFORNIA

Sara Levitt, a graduate student, was heavy her entire life. "Most of my family is overweight. It seemed that we were just prone to being larger people. But I always exercised. I figured that simply exercising would be enough and that I didn't have to watch what I ate because I was exercising regularly.

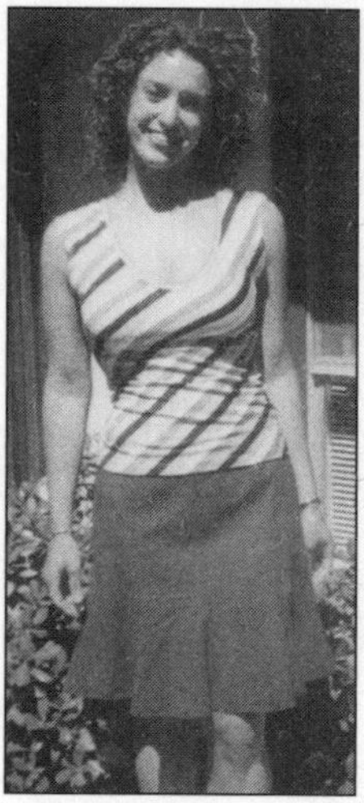

"My weight was always high and I never was happy or confident with the way I looked, but I figured that I was meant to be big. In my freshman year of college, I stopped exercising. Within a few months, I had reached my highest weight ever. One day, I just got tired of being unhappy with myself and thought that it was worth a try to make things different.

"I joined Weight Watchers. Then three close relatives died, including my father. It would have been so easy to go right back to my old habits out of stress and grief. But I remembered how much support I got from my father and knew that he would be disappointed if I didn't stick with it. So I did. Now I do activities that I never could have done before, like jogging and kick boxing. I am having so much fun that I hardly realize I am exercising."

*"Now I do activities that I never could have done before, like jogging and kick boxing."*

Sara lost 59 pounds to reach her goal weight. She recently wore a two-piece bathing suit for the first time since she was 9 years old and has a newfound confidence that has changed her life in countless positive ways.

calories in and calories out. You gain weight if you take in more calories than you burn, and you lose weight if you burn more calories than you take in.

To lose 1 pound, you need to create a calorie deficit of 3,500 calories. Over a week, this translates into 500 calories a day. You can create this calorie deficit through a combination of increased physical activity and cutting back on food. But how much can exercise contribute? Can it be an effective stand-alone weight-loss solution?

## Food Counts

Exercise alone as a weight-loss method is particularly ineffective without paying attention to food intake, and increasing activity is not a free pass to ignore eating habits. People who begin an exercise program often overlook the food side of the calories in/calories out equation. Some people even increase the amount of food they eat because they think they are burning more calories than they really are. The end result—weight gain rather than weight loss!

Going to the gym without a similar effort on the food front is sure to backfire. Numerous research studies show that it is common for people who are trying to lose weight to overestimate their physical activity—they think that they worked longer and harder than they really did. People also underestimate the amount of food or calories they are eating. So the difference between calories in from food and calories out from exercise is smaller than they think.

It is all too easy to overeat any time spent in exercise. For example, it takes about an hour on the treadmill for a 170-pound man to burn off a medium-size bagel (without butter or cream cheese), a few cookies, or a donut. A 150-pound woman doing a 30-minute workout at a circuit training gym like Curves burns about 150 calories, or the equivalent of a 12-ounce glass of orange juice. That's not a lot of food.

## It Takes a Lot of Exercise

Burning enough calories to lose weight takes quite a bit of exercise. It takes about 5½ calories of activity per pound of body weight for a person to maintain his or her current body weight. For an adult weighing

170 pounds, that is 925 to 950 calories in daily activity. To lose 1 pound of fat through exercise alone, a person needs to burn an *additional* 3,500 calories. So in order for that 170-pound adult to lose 2 pounds per week without making any dietary changes, he would need to continue doing everything that he is currently doing—plus walk an *additional* 10 miles per day (that is 70 miles a week). That is a lot of exercise and time! Needless to say, walking is still a very good idea, as this chapter will show.

If your goal is to lose weight by playing basketball, it will take more than five hours of active playing to lose a pound. It is extremely difficult to exercise enough on a consistent basis to lose even 1 pound of fat without making any changes to your diet.

**CALORIES BURNED BY A 170-POUND PERSON DOING 30 MINUTES OF COMMON ACTIVITIES**

| Activity | Calories Burned |
|---|---|
| Walking the dog | 168 |
| Jogging | 382 |
| Biking | 250 |
| Playing basketball | 230 |
| General household chores | 138 |

*Source:* Calorie Control Council (www.caloriecontrol.org).

You just learned that it takes a lot of exercise to burn a lot of calories.

## The Role of Exercise in Weight Loss

Mathematically you can design an exercise schedule for yourself that burns enough calories to lose 1 to 2 pounds a week. While this works on paper, the level of exercise commitment such a regimen requires is not sustainable for the vast majority of people, especially if it is started all at once. Several panels of experts have looked at all of the evidence and reached the conclusion that while exercise is extremely important, it does not lead to significant weight loss on its own.

This does not mean that it is a waste of time to exercise. Exercise is one of the healthiest things that you can do for yourself. Even a moderate activity like walking for thirty minutes every day at a comfortable pace will burn an additional 200 calories. True, this is not enough activity to cause a dramatic drop in your weight, but it *will* give your weight loss a boost. Additionally, the few hundred calories that are burned with regular physical activity compensate for adding a bit more food to the eating plan during weight loss. That can make the difference between a diet that feels as if it's depriving and a weight-loss program that is livable.

It is important to have realistic expectations about what exercise can and cannot do for weight loss. During the early days and weeks of weight loss, scheduling exercise is a way to help organize the day. About 200 to 300 calories burned during exercise can give weight loss a bit of a push. Exercise also helps boost mood and helps control stress, as noted earlier in the chapter. At a time when living a healthier lifestyle is foremost in your mind, physical activity can be a bright spot in the day.

*Have you ever heard . . .*

**"My weight isn't going down because now that I'm exercising, I am putting on muscle."**

It is possible that weight can stay the same during a weight-loss program because exercise builds muscle, and muscle weighs more than fat. But it is unlikely. Muscle takes up space differently in the body. So the muscle argument works, if the scale is not going down but you find yourself needing to buy smaller clothes. If your weight and your clothing are staying the same, though, either you are not building muscle, you are not exercising as hard as you think you are, or you are eating too much.

So watch out for the trap in thinking that exercise alone will be enough for weight loss—that is a setup for disappointment. People who expect a lot of weight loss from exercise alone may become so discouraged that they give up their goal of losing weight or stop exercising altogether.

## No Single Exercise Works Best

No single type of exercise or exercise program is right for everyone. Nor does one type of activity work better than others. Some people prefer to add more activity to their daily routine—taking the steps instead of the elevator, parking farther away, washing the kitchen floor by hand, using a hand mower, and other things—rather than doing planned, structured exercise. That is okay. One randomized, controlled weight-loss study found that women who participated in a structured activity regimen (in this case, aerobic exercise classes) had the same results as those who increased time and effort spent doing everyday chores.

Adopt a step-by-step approach, adding exercise slowly rather than trying to do too much too fast. Spend the first few weeks becoming comfortable with and mastering your new eating plan before tackling a formal approach to physical activity. During the early phase of weight loss, diet changes have a greater effect than activity changes do.

Start simple with an activity like walking. Once you have fully incorporated your walking program into your daily life, then consider other types of aerobic activity or strength training. Remember to check first with your doctor, then to get advice from a certified personal trainer or fitness professional who has experience working with overweight adults. Proper training and guidance along with a gradual increase in activity helps prevent injuries.

Think comprehensively. Exercise is only one component of an overall approach to sustainable weight loss. Your eating plan, mindset, behaviors, and encouragement from friends and family are also important. Support from people around you may offer an added boost and motivator even if you choose to do the exercise by yourself. Something

**PICKING THE RIGHT ACTIVITY FOR YOU**

| Choosing an Activity That Is | Pro | Con |
|---|---|---|
| Done alone rather than in a group | You can do it whenever it fits your schedule.<br>It doesn't matter how you look. | There is no social interaction.<br>There is a lack of accountability if you do not do it. |
| Done at home | It is less expensive than joining a gym.<br>You can do it whenever it fits your schedule. | There may be distractions and interruptions that keep you from doing the activity.<br>There is less opportunity for social interaction. |
| Done with an instructor | You are more likely to get encouragement.<br>Accountability is increased.<br>There is less chance of injury. | It is more expensive.<br>Time is not flexible. |
| Moderate intensity | This is the best balance between calorie burning and endurance. | There is less impact on cardiovascular health. |

as simple as having your spouse watch the kids while you go out for a walk after dinner can be a big help.

Most importantly, make it fun! Physical activity or an exercise class should be something that you look forward to every day. After all, it is a great way to relieve stress, relax, and do something just for you. Match the activities you choose to your personality and lifestyle.

## Walking Works

Walking is a terrific activity that can significantly contribute to sustainable weight loss. It is easy and just about everyone can do it. Most

## *Personal Triumph*

### Jennifer Crow

IOWA

Jennifer Crow tried everything out there. She had never been successful with weight loss. Although she'd heard about Weight Watchers, she thought that she could do it on her own. Jennifer admits that being accountable only to herself was not working. She was also tired of shopping and finding nothing that fit or looked good.

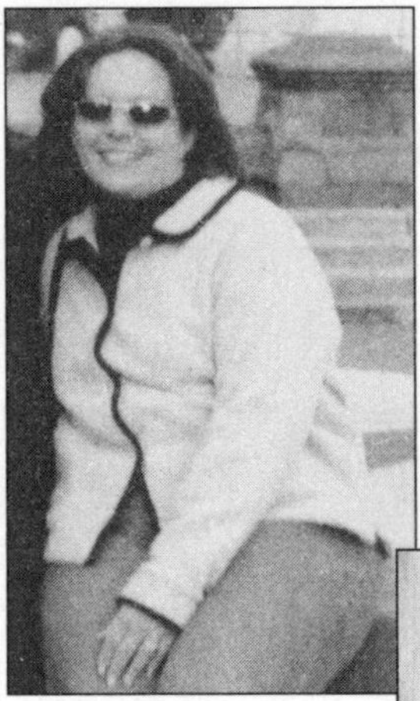

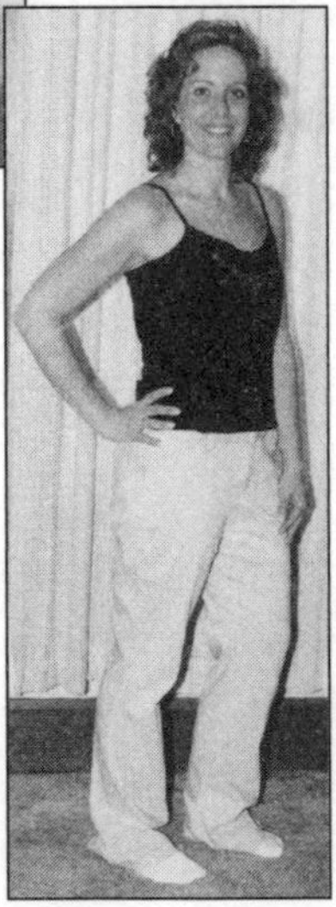

Jennifer joined Weight Watchers with the encouragement of a friend and started losing weight. That summer, she joined a softball team. "Now I work out five to six times a week after work, doing a combination of aerobics and aerobics with weight training in the comfort of my home. I credit my big boost in energy level to an increased commitment to exercise." She loves going up stairs without being out of breath and she no longer feels tired at the end of the day.

*"Now I work out five to six times a week after work."*

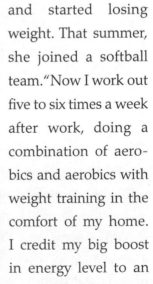

experts agree that walking is the preferred exercise for people who need to increase their physical activity as a part of their overall strategy for sustainable weight loss. Studies conducted at the Rippe Lifestyle Institute (RLI) have shown that starting regular walking programs can effectively boost weight loss, preserve lean muscle tissue, and improve mood. One study specifically looked at walking as part of a Weight Watchers program and found that regular walking was a highly effective component of a comprehensive weight-loss method.

Over 90% of NWCR participants say that they exercise almost every day. What is their preferred exercise? You guessed it, walking.

Walking has so many things going for it. It is a low-intensity exercise if you are strolling and a moderate-intensity exercise if done at a brisk pace. It does not cause a lot of pounding on bones and joints because one foot is always in contact with the ground during walking. Many other forms of exercise can be hard on the joints, especially with extra weight. Walking requires no special training or skill and can be done alone or with others. It does not require buying an expensive gym membership or exercise equipment. However, purchasing a good, sturdy pair of walking shoes can increase comfort and help avoid injury and blisters.

What's the best way to start a walking program? If you are just starting to get active, start slowly and build up slowly. It may take two or three months to reach a goal of thirty minutes per day, depending on your stamina. Choose a set time of day and schedule your walk in your calendar.

**Starting a Walking Program**

| | |
|---|---|
| Week 1 | 10 minutes per day |
| Week 2 | 12–13 minutes per day |
| Week 3 | 14–16 minutes per day |
| Week 4 | 16–19 minutes per day |
| Week 5 | 18–22 minutes per day |
| Week 6 on | Add 2–3 minutes per day each week |

People who have established a walking routine cannot imagine a day without the enjoyment of a regular walk.

## Moderate Intensity Is Best

The amount and intensity of activity determines its health benefits. Moderate-intensity exercise is recommended for weight loss and also improves your cardiovascular fitness. High-intensity exercise performed continuously for at least twenty minutes is recommended mainly for heart fitness. People who are more than 30 pounds overweight should not exercise at an intense level without talking to a doctor. Light activity burns only a modest amount of calories but offers numerous benefits. It generally does not burn enough calories to aid weight loss unless it is performed for a long period of time.

## Exercise Boosts Metabolism

Metabolism is a complex topic that we explore in detail in chapters 6 and 7. While specific diets and foods do not boost metabolism, exercise

**EXERCISE INTENSITY**

| Intensity | Types of Exercise | Physical Indicators | Benefits |
|---|---|---|---|
| Low | Leisurely walking, bicycling, swimming | Can talk and sing | Improves insulin sensitivity<br>Aids sleep<br>Boosts mood<br>Boosts confidence |
| Moderate | Brisk walking, bicycling, walking up stairs, gardening | Can carry on a conversation but cannot sing | Best balance among health benefits, calories spent, and exertion<br>Weight loss |
| High | Running, bicycle racing, competitive swimming | Can only speak in short phrases | Cardiovascular fitness |

does. Short term, there is increased energy burning during exercise. But the benefit extends beyond calorie burning. Regular exercise helps preserve lean body mass.

Lean body mass, also known as muscle, is the engine that drives the body's metabolism. Muscles work for the body every minute of every day, burning calories whether the body is sitting still, moving, or even sleeping. So if you preserve your lean body mass through physical activity, you get a double benefit—extra calorie burning during exercise and steady calorie burning throughout the day and night. Resistance training such as weight training, working with weight machines or bands, and even using your body as in a pushup preserves and builds muscle, muscle strength, and power, helping make daily tasks easier. You can stay active because your muscles are more fit.

Weight gain as we get older is common, but it is by no means inevitable. Adult weight gain does not result predominantly from a preprogrammed slowdown in metabolism that occurs with age—the main reason behind lower metabolism is an inactive lifestyle that causes lean muscle tissue to decrease. Here is the good news: you can build muscle and boost your metabolism no matter how old you are.

## Metabolic Effects

As with so many good things, the exercise–muscle–metabolism triangle has a few catches. Not all studies show that it is possible to preserve muscle mass during weight loss. The exact effect of exercise on the rate of metabolism, and therefore how many calories the body burns, is not consistent from person to person.

As weight goes down, the number of calories burned throughout the day and while doing a particular exercise also goes down because the muscles have less body weight to move around. Many aerobic exercise machines, like treadmills, step climbers, and elliptical machines, factor this in by including body weight in the estimate of the number of calories burned while on the machine.

The number of calories burned doing the same activity (for example, brisk walking for thirty minutes) decreases over time because the body gets into a groove and works more efficiently. Calorie burning also decreases over time as fitness level improves. Body movements become smoother and more coordinated.

To increase calories burned during exercise, increasing activity time is preferable to increasing activity intensity. Additionally, alternating activities can help prevent the muscles from getting too comfortable and efficient doing one particular form of exercise.

## Spot Training versus Aerobic Exercise

The myth of losing one's gut through abdominal exercises is part of a larger myth regarding "spot reduction." The common belief is that doing exercises specifically designed for one particular body part will reduce the fat in that area alone.

Scientific evidence shows that you cannot reduce fat in a specific area, like the abdomen, hips, or thighs, by doing exercises focused only on those areas. Toning specific sections of the body through spot and

*Have you ever heard . . .*

**"I will get rid of my gut by doing abdominal exercises."**

The desire for a flat stomach has spawned a multimillion-dollar industry of abdominal exercise machines. Who wouldn't want to look like the models featured in infomercials and advertisements? Unfortunately, using the latest and greatest abdominal machine will not build rock-hard abdominal muscles; nor will it develop a body builder's body. Muscles may get stronger by using spot toning equipment, but it takes much more to create the look you see in those ads. This is almost never achievable or sustainable for the average person with spot training alone.

strength training will, however, build muscles, make them look firmer, and even provide some change in their shape.

Spot or strength training is not very effective for losing overall body fat, either. Although this type of training builds muscle, giving the body a modest metabolic boost, it does not burn a lot of calories. The best exercise program combines the calorie-burning benefits of aerobic exercise—walking, cycling, swimming, jogging—with the toning benefits of strength training.

Start strength training slowly, especially if you have not been active or are not a consistent exerciser. Also, gradually add the strength training component of your fitness routine only after you have established a regular and consistent aerobic exercise program. This approach is highly effective.

## Exercise Helps Keep the Weight Off

Now let's learn how exercise can help prevent weight gain and also prevent regaining weight that has been lost. Numerous studies have shown that regular physical activity is one of the best predictors of weight maintenance. This factor is shared by a large majority of people who are successful at sustaining their weight loss.

Many, if not most, successful weight losers were not exercisers when they made the decision to lose weight. Rather, they began increasing their physical activity at some point during their weight-loss process. Over time, they came to enjoy the exercise itself and recognize the value it brings to sustaining their weight loss.

The amount of exercise connected with sustained weight loss is similar in most studies and surveys, and it is a significant amount. National Weight Control Registry (NWCR) participants report expending over 2,800 calories per week, or an average of 400 calories every day, doing physical activity. This is the equivalent of walking 4 miles a day. Another study found that 1,500 to 2,000 calories per week of exercise—walking roughly 15 to 20 miles over the course of the week—was associated with improved weight maintenance. Other researchers suggest that a formerly sedentary person needs eighty minutes of moderate activity (for example, brisk walking, dance aerobics) or thirty-five minutes of vigorous activity (for example, running, step aerobics) per day to minimize weight gain after weight loss. While the exact amounts of exercise differ somewhat, the message is clear: maintaining weight loss requires a commitment to exercise.

Regular physical activity has similar benefits when you're trying to keep the weight off as when you are trying to lose weight. It is a way to deal with stress and maintain a positive outlook. And it burns enough calories so that you can enjoy more food than you could otherwise eat while maintaining your weight.

### Fitness and Overweight

The relationship between overweight and physical fitness is a source of confusion and misinformation for many people. Some studies have found that a person's level of fitness has more impact on overall health and disease prevention than does excess body fat. While this is an interesting finding, the reality is that overweight and lack of fitness go together in the vast majority of people. Weight loss with a comprehensive method that includes regular physical activity provides the dual benefits of less body fat and improved fitness.

## The Bottom Line

Exercise is not an effective stand-alone weight-loss solution. Instead, regular exercise and increasing activity in your daily routine should be part of a well-rounded weight-loss program that includes smarter food choices, a positive frame of mind, and a supportive atmosphere. Together, they add up to positive changes in your lifestyle that you can live with to lose weight and keep it off.

Regular exercise is one of the most important things you can do to improve your health and well-being, as well as to achieve weight loss that lasts. Making small changes to your daily routine to increase your physical activity is an easy and effective strategy to help you manage your weight.

# Personal Triumph

## Joe Harasym

FLORIDA

Joe Harasym, whom we introduced in chapter 2, enjoyed walking outside when he lived in New York. Since retiring to Florida, he has even more opportunity to enjoy outdoor activities.

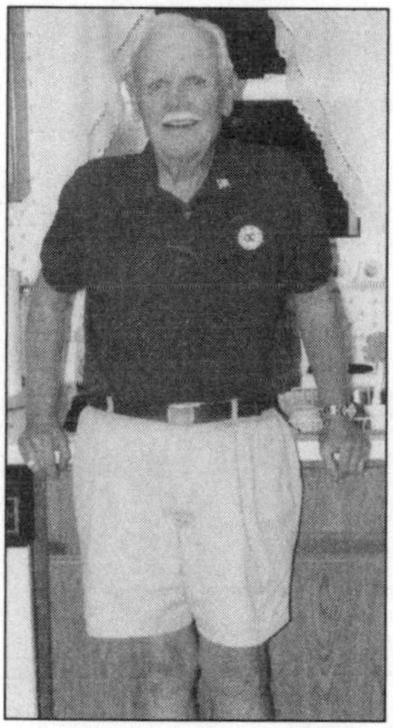

"While I have always been committed to exercise, I did not pay much attention to what I was eating until I joined Weight Watchers. I am a longtime walker, a couple of miles per day. That comes from when I was living and working in New York City. I always enjoyed walking but figured out that it wasn't enough because I gained weight. I thought I could lose weight by using a rowing machine, so I bought one. It was boring, even when I put it in front of the television.

*"Once I joined Weight Watchers, my entire commitment to eating and activity changed."*

"But once I joined Weight Watchers, my entire commitment to eating and activity changed. For example, my wife and I enjoy going on cruises. I found that even when on the ship, I can balance my eating and activity. On the last cruise that we took, I walked 2 or 3 miles every day around the ship's deck and enjoyed a lot of great meals."

## Weight Loss That Lasts

# Action Steps

Being physically active is a basic component in a comprehensive weight-loss method. Making exercise a part of your daily life can take time, but doing so is worth the effort. The benefits are many.

- Have realistic expectations for what exercise can and cannot do for you.
- Start slowly, maybe walking just ten minutes daily, and gradually build up from there.
- Choose an activity that fits into your lifestyle, that you enjoy, and that you can sustain.
- Schedule activity into your daily calendar.
- Include aerobic exercise to burn calories and strength training to tone and build your muscles.

# Chapter 5

# What counts the most—fats, carbs, or calories?

It seems it's always that one particular nutrient or type of food that has to be identified as the bad guy when it comes to weight and weight loss. In the 1960s and 1970s, we blamed overweight on breads and starchy foods, and thousands of people followed diets centered on meats, vegetables, and eggs. It was during this time that the popular coffee shop diet platter of a hamburger patty, cottage cheese, and half a canned peach was born. Then, in the 1990s, we blamed fat. Supermarket aisles quickly filled with fat-free foods as we rushed to siphon as much fat out of our diets as possible. Over the past few years, carbohydrates were put in the hot seat once again, and low-carbohydrate foods are taking the place of low-fat foods on the supermarket shelves.

In this chapter, you will learn about how the body uses fat and carbohydrates, and about which balance is best for losing weight and sustaining weight loss.

# Myth 5 Calories don't matter—avoid fats or carbs to lose weight successfully

*Believers Beware!*

Foods contain just three major nutrients—protein, fat, and carbohydrates. It is not the total amount of food people eat that causes them to gain weight. Rather, one of those big nutrients is playing havoc with the body. The key to weight loss is to eliminate foods that contain the one nutrient that causes weight gain. These days, following this strategy is possible since specialized foods that have reduced or eliminated the weight-causing nutrient are so widely available.

- Maybe fat is to blame. Fat in the diet is broken down into triglycerides that are taken in by body fat cells. Fat cells put triglycerides into storage and burn them very slowly and efficiently only after all other energy sources are used up. This works against weight loss. Eating fat also leads to heart attacks and cancer.
- Maybe carbohydrates (carbs) are the macronutrient that causes weight gain. Carbs make us fat because they force the body to overproduce the hormone insulin, the metabolism cop in the energy in/energy out equation that rules body weight. To keep blood sugar steady, insulin converts blood glucose from carbs into fat and pushes the fat into the fat cells. Insulin also prevents fat cells from releasing fat to be used for energy. Carbs make the body produce too much insulin, so blood sugar drops very fast. Since insulin will not let fat out to be used for energy, our brain tells us to eat more. If that food is a carb, the vicious cycle starts again. Eventually, the body becomes insulin resistant, and you gain weight. The answer is to eat very few carbohydrates. After cutting carbs, weight loss is quick and dramatic.
- Maybe it is protein. After all, vegetarians avoid animal-based protein for overall health and long-term weight management.

While the theories about the effects of fats and carbohydrates on weight are different, the myths are actually very similar. Let's take a closer look, starting with fat.

## Kernels of Truth

### Is Fat the Cause of Obesity and Poor Health?

Fat is very energy dense (more on energy density later). At 9 calories per gram, it supplies over twice the calories per gram of protein or carbohydrate. The number of calories in foods with fat adds up very quickly. Replacing fat with protein, or, more commonly, carbohydrate, can potentially cut down on calories.

Many popular foods contain a lot of fat. Baked desserts like cookies and cakes usually are loaded with fat, and so are snack foods and many restaurant foods. A survey conducted by the Institute of Food Technologists found that burgers, fries, Mexican food, and pizza—all packed with fat—are the most ordered foods in restaurants today.

Reducing fat intake can reduce calories and weight. Several years ago, people who were in a research study and following a low-fat diet for other reasons lost weight without even trying to lose it. Research literature now is quite clear on what happened: the low-fat diet was also lower in calories. Why? Food manufacturers had not yet created the hundreds of low-fat foods now available. Without the abundance of low-fat or fat-free cookies, ice cream, crackers, and other snacks and treats, dieters were left with basic food choices and not as much opportunity to overeat.

International studies that compared countries and research done on large groups of people have consistently shown a link between fat intake and obesity rates and between fat intake and diseases. Other studies have found that a diet low in fat, saturated fat, and cholesterol could reduce blood cholesterol levels and therefore lower the risk of heart disease. These findings have led the medical community to experiment with low-fat diets both to treat heart disease and to help people lose weight. It seems like good sense, since weight loss is one of the

# Personal Triumph

## Kathy Vollrath

ILLINOIS

Kathy Vollrath is a busy property manager who lost 104 pounds to reach her goal weight. Kathy tried to lose weight by cutting out fat, but it didn't work.

"I was thin through my 20s and then quickly became morbidly obese after my divorce at age 30. Every Monday I started something new—a different diet, pills, a hypnotist. Five years ago, my cholesterol was way over 300, I had high blood pressure and elevated triglyceride levels, and I was having chest pains. The doctor put me on medication to lower my cholesterol and gave me a low-fat diet. I decided to reduce my fat down to next to nothing, but I got constipated and didn't feel good.

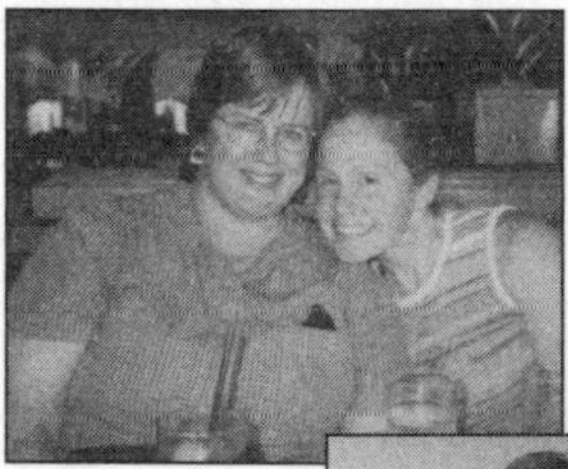

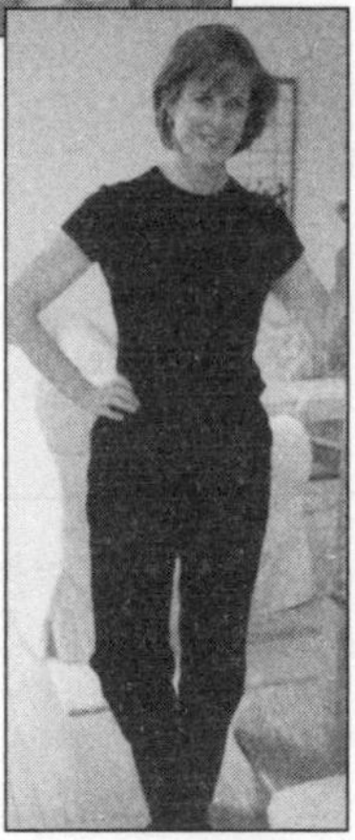

"One spring I was in a very serious accident and survived. I had a lot of time on my hands while I was lying in bed. I realized that I had been given a second chance and started thinking about life changes. I knew that I was obese and decided to do something about it. A woman at work was joining Weight Watchers and I asked if I could go with her to a meeting.

*"I'm an athlete now and I do triathlons with my daughter."*

"I'm an athlete now and I do triathlons with my daughter. My diet is balanced and I make sure that I eat healthy fats. I would not even consider cutting carbohydrates. The only way to lose weight and keep it off is to eat the right amount of food."

most powerful ways to lower heart disease risk. In cardiology circles, this was called the "diet heart hypothesis." Lowering the amount of fat in the diet could lower blood cholesterol and aid weight loss.

Different types of dietary fat have links to heart disease and cancer. A diet rich in *saturated fat,* a hard fat primarily in meats and dairy fat, increases heart disease risk, the number one killer of both men and women in our society. Saturated fat has also been linked to a higher risk of breast, prostate, and other cancers.

*Trans fat* is created in vegetable oil through hydrogenation to make the oil hard, similar to saturated fat. This is how margarines are made. Like saturated fat, trans fat increases blood cholesterol levels.

Some studies suggest that eating a lot of vegetable oils that are rich in omega-6 fatty acids (polyunsaturated fat) to the exclusion of other fats, thus creating an imbalance in the mix of fats, may contribute to some forms of cancer.

Ultimately, fat is fat—fat in the diet and fat on the body are the same. The message is simple: eat less fat and have less body fat.

## The Whole Truth

### Fat in Foods Is Important

Fat serves vital purposes in the diet because it contains several important vitamins and aids the absorption of other essential nutrients, including essential fatty acids, carotenoids, and fat-soluble vitamins. Fat in foods stimulates the gallbladder to contract as the food from a meal reaches the intestines. The bile that the gallbladder squirts into the digestive tract is needed to digest and absorb food.

The body requires fat from foods in order to function properly. In its most recent report, the Institute of Medicine (IOM) recommended that 20% to 35% of daily calories come from fat. For the first time, it also recommended specific amounts of two essential fatty acids: linoleic acid, an omega-6 fatty acid in vegetable oils, and alpha-linolenic acid, an omega-3 fatty acid in fatty fish. These fats are considered essential because the body is unable to produce them on its own.

**FAT-CONTAINING NUTRIENTS ESSENTIAL FOR GOOD HEALTH**

| Nutrients | Essential Fatty Acids | Fat-Soluble Vitamins | Carotenoids |
|---|---|---|---|
| Examples | Linoleic, alpha-linolenic | Vitamins A, D, E, K | Beta-carotene, lycopene, lutein |
| What They Do | Involved in regulating the body's inflammation, blood clotting, and cholesterol systems | Involved in all body functions, but particularly in tissues like the bones, eyes, blood, and skin; vitamin E is an antioxidant | Antioxidants—substances that work against the breakdown in body functions linked with the development of conditions like heart disease |
| Good Sources | Nuts, grains, seeds, some oils | Eggs, whole grains, nuts, oils, meat and fatty fish, vegetables that are colorful (e.g., red, orange, dark green) | Fruits and vegetables that are colorful (e.g., red, orange, dark green) |

In recent years, a great deal has been learned about fat. Different kinds serve different functions in the body, and it is often the balance between fats that makes the difference. The Mediterranean diet is an example of a higher-fat but balanced-fat diet. People who eat the Mediterranean-style diet of fruits, vegetables, fish, legumes, breads and cereals, and olive oil have a lower risk of heart disease and certain cancers. The actual amount of fat eaten in a Mediterranean diet is not low, but it is associated with positive health at least in part because of the mix of the fats it contains.

With this new understanding about the role of fats in health, in the most recent edition of the *Dietary Reference Intakes,* the IOM liberalized its recommendation of the percent of fat in a balanced diet. The maximum recommended percentage of calories coming from fat was increased from 30% to 35%. This revised recommendation gives greater flexibility for eating more fat in the diet, provided the fats one eats include more unsaturated sources. Eating more saturated or trans fats is never recommended for good health.

Eating too little fat can cause problems. A very low-fat diet does not stimulate the gallbladder to contract and empty its bile, increasing the risk of gallstone formation. Most very low-fat diets are high in carbohydrates. A high-carbohydrate diet can increase triglycerides in some people. For this reason, very low-fat diets for weight loss are not recommended by either the American Heart Association or the American Diabetes Association. Very low-fat diets are too low in several nutrients, including vitamin E. This is particularly noteworthy because the increasing need for this vital nutrient has been recognized for its role as an antioxidant. The latest edition of the *Dietary Reference Intakes* increased the recommended daily amount of vitamin E from 8 milligrams for women and 10 milligrams for men to 15 milligrams for both men and women.

## There Are No Free Foods, Part I

Fat-free foods are not free foods. When people eat processed low-fat and fat-free foods in large or unlimited amounts under the misconception that calories do not matter, they don't lose weight. In fact, they gain weight. The United States has experienced a shocking increase in the amount and severity of obesity over the past thirty years during the very time that low-fat foods have exploded in the marketplace.

It is easy to completely replace calories from high-fat foods with fat-free, high-carbohydrate, high-sugar foods with just as many calories. Many people even eat larger portions of fat-free cookies because they have no fat. Weight loss occurs only when you eat fewer calories, not when daily calories stay the same.

Thousands of foods with little to no nutritional or weight-loss value were developed and sold during the height of the low-fat craze. Food companies made millions, and shoppers eagerly awaited the next new product. Many people were disappointed as they ate more of these specialty foods with an expectation of weight loss only to gain weight. This is often referred to as "Snackwells Syndrome" after the popular line of cookies that was marketed as low-fat.

## The Truth about Fat—Balance Is Best

The optimal diet for weight loss and sustaining weight loss is neither high nor very low in fat. The optimal diet is a balanced one. A balanced diet meets the IOM recommendation of 20% to 35% of calories from fat. Generally, diets that derive 20% to 30% of their calories from fat are considered low in fat. Some popular low-fat diets actually are *very* low-fat diets, with fat limited to less than 10% of calories. Balanced diets supply up to 35% of calories from fat and include diets like the Mediterranean diet and DASH, a diet high in fruits and vegetables and low-fat dairy products designed by government researchers to help reduce high blood pressure. Shifting from a high-fat diet to a balanced diet can assist in weight loss because total calories are lowered.

All fats have the same number of calories, so they have the same effect on body weight. However, the types and ratios of fats eaten are important for health. The table on the following page summarizes some of the information about fats and their known or suggested health consequences. As you can see, not all fats are created equal.

Saturated fat and trans fat should be limited because they can raise total blood cholesterol levels and lower levels of good HDL cholesterol. Saturated fat is hard fat found primarily in red meat and full-fat dairy products. Trans fat helps add crispiness to cookies, crackers, doughnuts, breaded foods, and other baked or fried foods. When food manufacturers tried to decrease saturated fat in their products, they turned to trans fat, creating unanticipated health problems comparable to those associated with saturated fat. Many food manufacturers are now removing all or most of the trans fat from their products, and the Nutrition Facts label is being revised to include trans fat information.

Polyunsaturated fats can be included in moderation. They help lower blood cholesterol when they are substituted for saturated fat in

**COMPARING FATS**

| Primary Type of Fat | Found in | Health Effects |
|---|---|---|
| Saturated | Cheese, butter, whole milk, meat and meat fat, cocoa butter, coconut and palm oils | Raises blood cholesterol |
| Trans | Fried chicken, doughnuts, cookies, crackers, baked goods | Raises blood cholesterol |
| Polyunsaturated | Soft margarine, vegetable oils | Lowers blood cholesterol when substituted for saturated fat, may lower HDL<br>Increased cancer risk if consumed in large amounts |
| Monounsaturated | Chicken, fish, olive and canola oils, nuts, avocados | Lowers blood cholesterol, maintains HDL |
| Omega-3 | Fish, flaxseed | Lowers risk of heart disease and sudden death |

the diet. Unfortunately, sometimes they lower beneficial HDL cholesterol along with total cholesterol. Polyunsaturated fats are a rich source of vitamin E in the diet.

Two types of fats are extremely beneficial: monounsaturated fats and omega-3 fats. Monounsaturated fats, such as those in olive oil, canola oil, and many nuts, help lower total cholesterol. An added benefit is that they preserve or even raise levels of HDL cholesterol. The omega-3 fatty acids in many types of deep-sea fish, including salmon, mackerel, and bluefish, have been shown to lower the risk of both heart disease and sudden death. Including at least 2 teaspoons per day of a healthy oil (for example, canola, olive, safflower, sunflower, flaxseed) can go a long way in creating the right ratio of fatty acids. Fortunately, these oils are very versatile and provide a nice added touch to your eating plan. They can be used as a salad dressing, as a spread on bread, or to season or sauté vegetables.

### Fat Adds Food Flexibility

Having a balanced approach to fat may actually aid in weight loss. Researchers in Boston compared two groups of people who were prescribed weight-loss diets that varied in their fat content. The group whose diet included more fat (35% of total calories, with the extra fat coming from olive oil and other monounsaturated fats) had fewer people drop out of the study. This group also ate more vegetables, possibly because adding a small amount of fat to vegetables and salads makes them taste better.

### Lower-Energy-Density Foods

Lower-fat foods are often low-energy-density foods, meaning that they are higher in water and not very concentrated in calories. Reducing the energy density of the diet reduces calories without unduly limiting the amount of food that is eaten. If your diet is based on the less-energy-dense foods that are typically consumed on a balanced diet, you may have the sensation that you are eating more food while losing weight. The experience of the Rippe Lifestyle Institute (RLI) has been that people following a diet that is lower in fat than what they were eating before coming to the institute say that they never feel deprived or hungry.

**Lower- versus Higher-Energy Density**

Calories add up much more slowly if you choose foods that are naturally low in fat and low in energy density. Each food listed below supplies 100 calories.

| *Lower-Energy Density* | *Higher-Energy Density* |
|---|---|
| 1⅓ cups chicken noodle soup | ½ cup tomato bisque |
| 2 cups cantaloupe chunks | 12 potato chips |
| 18 large steamed shrimp | 1½ slices hard salami |
| 2¼ cups puffed wheat cereal | 1 mini-croissant |

Make no mistake about it—calories count, so watch out! It is very possible to eat a low-fat, lower-energy-density food, slather butter, olive oil, or a high-fat salad dressing on it, and turn it into a high-fat, high-calorie food. In fact, many of the fast-food salads topped with regular dressing have more fat and calories than a fast-food burger.

### Balance Makes Sense

Very low-fat diets often don't work long term because people go back to their old eating habits. As people slip back into their previous way of eating, the weight comes back. In contrast, a diet balanced with respect to fat is closely linked with sustained weight loss.

A balanced diet encourages and allows food choices from all the major food groups, creating a very healthy and nutritionally sound food pattern. Very low-fat diets may fall short in key nutrients. The more restricted the diet, the more difficult it is to meet all recommendations for vitamins and minerals.

Now, let's take a closer look at carbohydrates.

## Kernels of Truth

### Are Carbohydrates the Cause of Obesity and Poor Health?

According to data from the Continuing Survey of Food Intakes of Individuals (CSFII), a survey of a representative sampling of Americans, the amount of carbohydrates in the American diet and the percent of calories from carbohydrates have increased over the past twenty years. During this time, calories have also gone up by about 300 per day and the percent of calories from fat have decreased from about 40% to about 34%. The biggest increases have been from sweetened beverages like soda and fruit juices and from carbohydrate-containing mixed-grain dishes like pizza and tacos.

"Reducing carbohydrates lowers calories, and that means weight loss." This observation dates back to 1860, when an Englishman, William Banting, claimed that he lost 46 of his initial 202 pounds by cutting out carbohydrates. Banting wrote, "The great charms and

# *Personal Triumph*

## Gerry Smart

MINNESOTA

*"A friend was going to Weight Watchers and I asked if I could come with her to a meeting. I went, joined, and found out that Weight Watchers was just what I needed."*

Gerry Smart always had a lot of pounds to lose, and she lost them and gained them back many times over. Gerry and her family moved frequently—just as she settled in to a new hometown, it was time to move again.

"I gained weight every time I moved because I was lonesome and turned to food. Then I would try to lose weight. You name the diet, I tried it. I lost weight every time, no matter what diet it was.

"I've been on several different low-carb diets, but I didn't feel right when I was on them—I was dizzy all the time. Of course, after I lost weight, I gained it back a little bit at a time. At one point I even decided that I should just be happy with my weight where it was.

"When I moved to my current home in Minnesota, I wanted that cycle of losing and regaining to stop. Also, I had back pain, knee pain, high blood pressure, terrible heartburn, and constant fatigue—I felt lousy. It was time to do something. A friend was going to Weight Watchers and I asked if I could come with her to a meeting. I went, joined, and found out that Weight Watchers was just what I needed."

Gerry joined Weight Watchers about two years ago and is maintaining her goal weight loss of 104 pounds!

comfort of this system are that its effects are palpable within a week of trial and creates a natural stimulus to persevere for a few weeks more." Needless to say, Banting gained back the weight he lost! Any diet that restricts major food groups and therefore cuts out a major nutrient—carbohydrate, fat, or protein—will cut calories and result in short-term weight loss but not for the long term.

The way that carbohydrates are stored and processed in the body is different from that for fats. Insulin plays an important role in the metabolism of carbohydrates. The body produces insulin in a finely regulated way to manage the inflow of blood sugar after eating. Carbohydrates act like a sponge in the body. Every gram of carbohydrate that is stored in the body as glycogen, a type of carbohydrate the body uses to meet short-term energy needs, holds on to an additional 3 grams of water. When the body uses up glycogen, it also releases water and extra weight. This phenomenon creates the illusion of a quick loss of body fat.

## The Whole Truth

### Carbohydrates Are Essential

Carbohydrates in the form of a sugar called glucose are the preferred source of energy by the body. Any source of carbohydrates except fiber can be converted into glucose by the body. This conversion process is a fundamental part of the digestion and metabolism of food. For some parts of the body, including the brain, glucose is the only fuel source that can be used to meet energy needs. The need for glucose is so important to our survival that, when deprived of carbohydrates, the body will take extreme metabolic actions to manufacture the glucose that it needs. It has systems in place that, if required, can take the protein out of muscle, strip off the nitrogen bits that make it a protein, and convert the rest to glucose. Over time this process is quite detrimental, potentially resulting in a buildup of nitrogen that leads to the development of kidney stones or gout. The body will sacrifice muscle for glucose in order to survive.

Based on a complete review of the human need for glucose, the Institute of Medicine (IOM) has set the Recommended Daily Allowance for carbohydrates at a minimum of 130 grams per day. Following an extreme diet that restricts carbohydrates to less than 130 grams per day means that the body must resort to survival systems to make its own glucose, usually at the cost of muscle, to meet its minimal needs. Many extreme low-carb diets require that you eat no more than 20 grams of carbohydrates per day. To put that into perspective, a cup of milk has 12 grams of carbohydrates, a slice of regular bread has 15 grams, and a large apple has 20 grams.

## Carb-Rich Foods Are Often Nutritious

In addition to being the body's preferred source of energy, foods rich in carbohydrates contain several essential nutrients that are important for nutritional health and disease prevention. Wholesome carbohydrate foods like fruits, vegetables, grains, and legumes supply fiber, vitamins, and minerals. Low-fat dairy foods like milk and yogurt are rich in carbohydrates and are also important sources of calcium, vitamin D, zinc, and protein. Avoiding carbohydrate-rich foods can lead to shortfalls of these essential nutrients. Each food group supplies different combinations of macronutrients (carbohydrates, proteins, fats, fiber, and water), vitamins, and minerals. A nutritionally sound diet contains foods from all the food groups.

Beyond meeting basic nutritional needs, making food choices that include a wide variety of wholesome carbohydrate-rich foods has consistently been shown to lead to a reduced risk for many chronic diseases, including high blood pressure, kidney disease, osteoporosis, heart disease, and several forms of cancer. The mechanisms by which these foods prevent disease are numerous. Many of the specifics have not yet been discovered, but more is being learned every day. For example, it is known that fruits, vegetables, and whole grains are rich in phytochemicals. These compounds, which include thousands of substances produced naturally by plants, lower the risk of developing various forms of cancer. Low-fat dairy foods, a great source of calcium, are linked with a reduced risk of osteoporosis. And fruits, vegetables, dairy products, and whole grains are all good sources of potassium, a mineral linked with preventing high blood pressure.

**CARB-CONTAINING NUTRIENTS ESSENTIAL FOR GOOD HEALTH**

| Nutrients | Fiber | Vitamins | Minerals |
|---|---|---|---|
| Examples | Soluble, insoluble | B vitamins, vitamin C, folic acid | Calcium, potassium, magnesium |
| What They Do | Regulate bowel function and cholesterol removal from the body | Prevent deficiencies and work as antioxidants | Serve as catalysts for all the chemical reactions needed for life |
| Good Sources | Whole grains, dried beans and legumes, fruits and vegetables | Whole grains, enriched grain products, fruits and vegetables | Low-fat dairy foods, whole grains, fruits and vegetables |

## Not All Carbs Are Created Equal

Carbohydrates are classified into three groups: sugars, starches, and fiber. Sugars include sucrose (table sugar), fructose (fruit sugar), lactose (milk sugar), syrup, honey, and other caloric sweeteners. Fruits and some vegetables contain sugars, which are easily digested and absorbed into the body. Starches are present in breads, cereals, grains, potatoes, peas, and many other vegetables. They take longer to digest and are absorbed into the body more slowly. Most fiber is nondigestible and never turns into blood sugar. Fiber in foods does not contribute calories. Whole grains, legumes (dried peas and beans), vegetables, and fruits supply fiber.

The types of carbohydrate-containing foods in the diet matter. Sugars and starches have the same number of calories and the same effect on body weight. However, the foods from which they are eaten have varied nutrition profiles—high-sugar foods tend to be less nutritious

**Healthy Carbohydrate Picks**

- Whole grains and whole-grain products
- Fruits
- Vegetables
- Low-fat dairy products

than foods with less sugar. The IOM recommends that no more than 25% of calories come from added sugar in foods and in the form of caloric sweeteners like sugar and honey. For most people, especially those who are working to lose weight, this means minimizing sugar-containing beverages like soda, sweetened iced tea, and other sweetened drinks, sugary desserts like ice cream and cookies, and other highly sweetened foods.

Several other types of carbohydrate-containing foods are important. Whole grains are preferable to processed grains. They are rich in fiber as well as starch and often provide more nutrients than their processed counterpart. For example, brown rice supplies more fiber and minerals than white rice. Whole grains also improve eating satisfaction. Fruits and vegetables supply phytochemicals, fiber, vitamins, and minerals. Most are low-energy-density foods that are naturally low in fat and higher in fiber. Low-fat dairy foods like nonfat milk and yogurt offer a rich array of important nutrients like calcium and protein.

## The Truth about Carbs—Balance Is Best

The optimal diet for losing weight and keeping it off is neither high nor low in carbohydrates. What is a balanced diet? The IOM recommends that 45% to 65% of calories come from carbohydrates. Recommended intakes of fiber are 38 grams per day for adult men and 25 grams per day for adult women. Meeting this fiber recommendation, especially when calories are being reduced to lose weight, means making wise food choices that include whole grains and cereals, dried beans and legumes, and whole fruits and vegetables.

# Personal Triumph

## Michelle Krischke

TEXAS

Michelle Krischke, whom we met in chapter 3, tried many different weight-loss methods before joining Weight Watchers. She lost weight on all of them, but because she did not learn how to eat, she just followed rules about what not to eat and her weight came right back once she returned to her old eating habits. Then she was diagnosed with two herniated disks and decided to lose weight quickly.

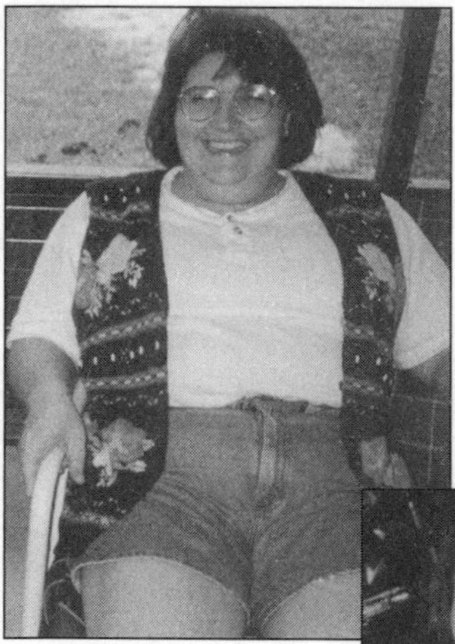

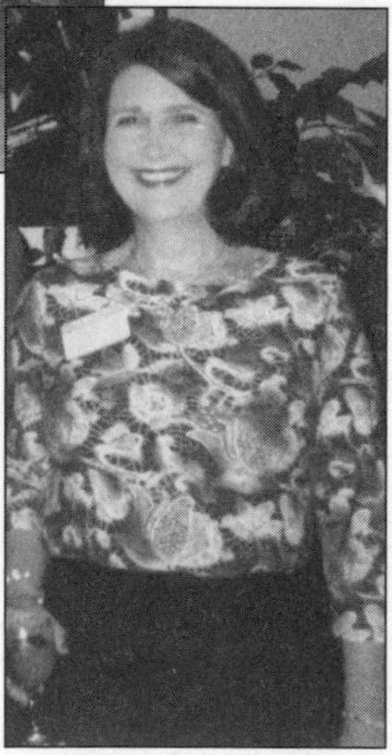

*“Today, I understand the role of carbohydrates in my diet and enjoy a slice of pizza on occasion.”*

“I picked up a low-carbohydrate diet book from the bookstore, along with a large pizza from the pizzeria, and went home to read the book and learn about foods to avoid, including pizza! Today, I understand the role of carbohydrates in my diet and enjoy a slice of pizza on occasion.”

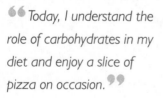

A balanced diet that includes wholesome, nutritious, carbohydrate-rich foods is closely linked with sustained weight loss. Merely shifting from a diet that includes a lot of added sugars and refined starches to one that is rich in whole grains, fruits, and vegetables can assist in weight loss by offering eating satisfaction from foods that are filling and lower in calories. Foods like fresh fruits and vegetables that have lower energy density help reduce calories without unduly limiting the amount of food that is eaten. The calorie deficit necessary for weight loss is created without a sacrifice to nutritional health and well-being.

## There Are No Free Foods, Part 2

Some diets and food products use the terms *net carbs, effective carbs,* and *impact carbs*. These terms, which we will simply call *adjusted carbs,* were created by food marketers in an effort to make their foods appeal to people following a low-carb diet. There currently are no recognized legal or scientific definitions for adjusted carbs, but most food manufacturers calculate the number by subtracting dietary fiber and sugar alcohols (see below) from the total carbohydrates. Because they have been created and are being used extensively to sell foods, the Food and Drug Administration (FDA) is considering their use.

The theory behind adjusted carbs has to do with the way carbohydrates are digested and metabolized in the body. Fiber is not absorbed in digestion, so it does not turn into glucose. Sugar alcohols—sorbitol, mannitol, maltitol, and other ingredients that end in *-ol*—are food ingredients that are used as sweeteners. They are carbohydrate/alcohol mixes that are metabolized more slowly than starches and sugars. This slower digestion means less impact on the blood sugar level than traditional carbohydrate-rich foods. Sugar alcohols contain calories, which are calories used as an energy source by the body. To date, no single scientific study has demonstrated that using foods based on their adjusted carbs results in weight loss.

Food manufacturers have created thousands of low-carbohydrate alternatives to traditional higher-carbohydrate processed foods. Pasta, bread, cereal, ice cream, cookies, candy, and even beer are now available in reduced-carbohydrate versions. The carbohydrates that are removed have to be replaced with something, and sugar alcohols or protein isolates from soy are the most frequently used replacements. Sugar alcohols have a laxative effect and can cause gas, bloating, stomach pain, and diarrhea in many people.

Proteins and carbohydrates each have 4 calories per gram. Sugar alcohols have 5 calories per gram (though not all are usable by the body). A food product that substitutes protein or a sugar alcohol for carbohydrates does not offer savings in terms of calories per serving. The likelihood of losing weight by substituting low-carb versions of favorite foods for their traditional counterparts is nil because calories are not reduced.

When it comes to weight management, calories are calories,

*Have you ever heard . . .*

**Have you ever heard . . . "Sugar substitutes, like aspartame, sucralose, and saccharine, actually make you gain weight."**

Despite a great deal of rumor to the contrary, there is no scientific evidence that the use of these products is linked with weight gain. In theory, use of these products should produce weight loss because of the calorie savings from substituting a no-calorie sweetener for a calorie-containing sugar. The reality, however, is that most studies do not show an effect—positive or negative—between weight and their use. Most experts believe that people compensate for the calorie savings by choosing to eat more calorie-containing foods. In a recent study on the topic, the subjects were more influenced by how many calories they thought they were eating than by whether the food actually contained sugar or a substitute.

and eating too many calories regardless of the source will lead to weight gain.

## The Role of Insulin

The theory behind low-carb weight-loss diets focuses on insulin and its role in the body. There is a kernel of truth in the theory because insulin is intimately involved in the metabolism of glucose. However, the pancreas produces insulin in a finely regulated way to manage the inflow of blood glucose after a meal and to help manage the daily ups and downs of blood glucose. Even when blood sugar goes up significantly after a meal, most bodies do not produce excess insulin. Hypoglycemia and diabetes, two conditions related to insulin, are serious medical conditions.

Hypoglycemia, which literally means low levels of glucose in the blood, can be caused by liver disease, surgical absence of the stomach, tumors that release excess amounts of insulin, and prediabetes. While many people believe that they have hypoglycemia, a true medical diagnosis is relatively rare, requiring that the person have symptoms (anxiety, sweating, tremor, palpitations, nausea, and pallor) with a documented blood glucose level of less than 45 mg/dl, and there must be complete resolution of the symptoms with the administration of glucose.

The treatment for hypoglycemia requires identification of the underlying cause. For people who have hypoglycemia as part of the early development of diabetes, dietary recommendations include a consistent intake of total carbohydrates from day to day and eating smaller meals spaced throughout the day.

Diabetes, or diabetes mellitus, is a group of metabolic diseases that result from defects in the way insulin is produced, used by the body, or both. The hallmark of diabetes is high levels of glucose in the blood. There are two major types of diabetes mellitus, called type 1 and type 2. In type 1 diabetes mellitus, the pancreas stops making insulin. A patient with type 1 diabetes must rely on insulin medication for survival. About 10% of people with diabetes have type 1; 90% have type 2.

In type 2 diabetes, the pancreas still produces insulin but inadequately. In many cases, the pancreas produces larger than normal quantities of insulin, but the body's cells do not react to it correctly. This is known as insulin resistance.

The treatment for diabetes focuses on the maintenance of blood glucose levels within a desirable range. Type 1 diabetes is treated with insulin, exercise, and a diabetic diet. Type 2 diabetes is treated with weight reduction, a diabetic diet, and exercise. When these measures fail to control the elevated blood glucose levels, medications are used.

Adherence to a diabetic diet is an important aspect of controlling diabetes. The American Diabetes Association (ADA) has provided guidelines for a diabetic diet. The ADA diet is balanced in both fat and carbohydrate intake. Fruits, vegetables, low-fat dairy foods, and wholesome grains are all important. Sugar and sugar-containing foods can be eaten as part of a healthy, balanced diet for diabetes.

There is a strong link between excess weight and the risk of developing diabetes. The fact is, though, that most overweight people do not have diabetes and are able to produce and process insulin normally.

## Beyond Insulin

In addition to insulin, the body produces a large number of other hormones that work together to tightly control the flow of energy systems in the body. The human body is a marvel at creating systems of checks and balances to ensure survival. The need for a steady source of glucose to the brain is too important for the body to rely on a single hormone like insulin. There is a cascade of hormones and related compounds that work together at all times to ensure that there is not too little or too much glucose circulating in the body.

Another key hormone that regulates blood sugar is called *glucagon*. This hormone is the counterpart to insulin and is released when blood sugar starts to get low. Glucagon signals the body to release some of its stored glycogen into the blood to keep blood glucose levels steady. This finely tuned system prevents the roller-coaster effect that insulin could have if it existed alone and helps to explain why wide swings in blood sugar are rare. People who have these swings require intense medical care.

But using stored glycogen has an effect on weight loss because it provides only 4 calories per gram (fat supplies 9 calories per gram) and a glycogen molecule is about 75% water. Eliminating carbohydrates forces the body to dip into its reserves of glycogen. As the body pulls from these reserves, the glycogen sponge is squeezed and water is released with the glucose that is stored as glycogen, leading to a temporary weight loss from water loss.

Low-carbohydrate diets lead to significant early weight loss. But the pounds lost are not all fat. A significant portion of this weight loss is water loss, which the body ultimately recovers. Some studies suggest that as much as half of the initial weight loss on a low-carbohydrate, high-fat diet is water loss. In essence, following this type of diet is like taking a diuretic because the body is forced to get rid of a lot of water very quickly. And the weight loss does not last.

Eliminating carbs means eating more of something else to make up for the missing calories. While most people assume that a low-carbohydrate diet is high in protein, many studies have found otherwise. Indeed, people following this diet tend to increase their protein intake only moderately. Most animal sources of protein—meat, poultry, cheese, and eggs—supply both protein and fat. People on low-carbohydrate diets get some of their calories from animal protein sources; the rest comes from added fats like butter and oils. That is why the major increase in low-carbohydrate diets is in fat intake—following a low-carb diet is really following a high-fat diet for most people.

Because diets that eliminate or severely restrict carbohydrates are so extreme, they are difficult to sustain. Virtually all of the studies that have looked at following a low-carb diet for more than a few months have found that the early weight loss is not sustained. Researchers state that these diets cannot be followed for more than short periods of time because they are so restrictive and require high levels of dietary

# *Personal Triumph*

## Alan Weinstein

CALIFORNIA

Alan Weinstein, a business owner, struggled with his weight for many years. Then an accident injured his knees, causing his weight to skyrocket to over 300 pounds. Low-carb diets helped him lose weight, but he could not keep the weight off.

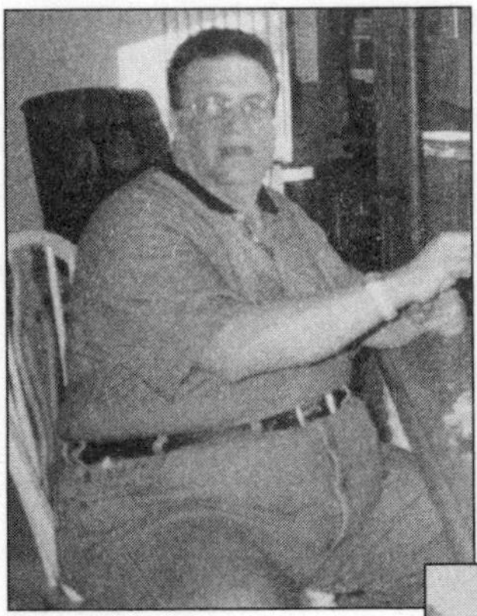

"I needed something that I could live with and stay with. My daughter encouraged me to join Weight Watchers, and my wife, a Lifetime Member, said that she would go to meetings with me.

"When I joined Weight Watchers, I weighed 329 pounds, was in the early stages of developing diabetes, and had high blood pressure and an elevated cholesterol level. Weight Watchers helped me become more aware of what I was eating and what it was doing to me. Now that I'm so aware of my eating habits, I go right back to habits that will maintain my weight. That's the difference. With the old way of dieting, my weight went up and down, then up and up and up."

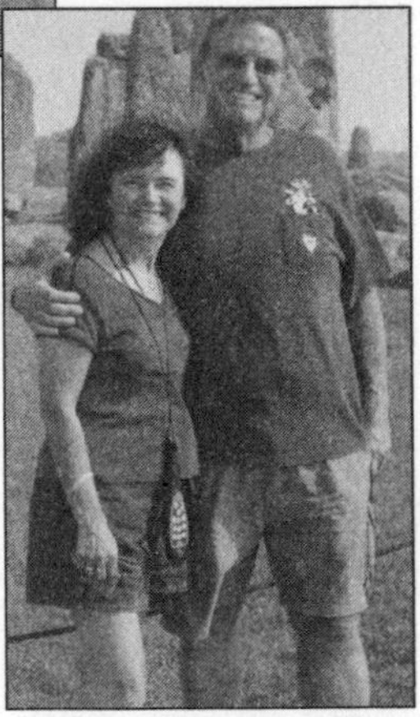

*"Weight Watchers helped me become more aware of what I was eating and what it was doing to me."*

Not any more. Alan lost over 105 pounds to reach his goal weight.

restraint. It goes without saying that weight loss only occurs as long as the lower-calorie eating plan is continued, and weight loss cannot be sustained if the eating plan is not adopted as part of a long-term lifestyle change.

## The Bottom Line

A balanced diet that supplies a healthy ratio of fats along with nutritious carbohydrates can aid weight loss and long-term weight maintenance. This type of diet includes all the food groups and supplies essential, health-promoting nutrients in amounts recommended by government agencies and health organizations. A balanced diet contains appropriate amounts of fats for heart health along with recommended levels of fiber.

Both fats and carbohydrates are essential nutrients. In addition, foods that are good sources of these macronutrients provide other essential nutrients like vitamins, minerals, essential fatty acids, and phytochemicals that prevent nutritional deficiencies and reduce the risk of developing several diseases.

For both fats and carbs, there are better and not-so-great food choices. The key is to make wise food choices without resorting to an extreme diet. This can be done with an eating style of flexible restraint that emphasizes nutrient-packed, low-energy-density foods that provide eating satisfaction.

Information in the two major databases of large groups of people who have lost weight and kept it off, the Weight Watchers LTM survey and the National Weight Control Registry (NWCR) participants, suggests that a balanced diet that includes the recommended levels of fat and carbohydrates can be sustained successfully. NWCR participants also report eating breakfast on most days of the week, with cereal—a high-carbohydrate food—as the most popular breakfast choice. The Weight Watchers program is designed to be a balanced diet that includes wholesome foods like healthy oils, fruits and vegetables, milk and milk products, and whole grains.

## Weight Loss That Lasts

# Action Steps

Food, weight, and health are intricately interwoven. To keep the balance between them, the best approach is a balanced diet. When you cut out a macronutrient, you eliminate the essential nutrients and potential health benefits that may come with it. Here are things that you can do to optimize your balanced diet:

- Select foods with healthier fats—monounsaturated, polyunsaturated, and omega-3 fats—and include them in your diet when you will enjoy them most.
- Reduce the saturated fats in your diet by choosing lean meats and lower-fat dairy products.
- Reduce the trans fats in your diet by limiting doughnuts, fried chicken, crackers, cookies, and other baked goods. Check ingredient lists for the presence of partially hydrogenated oil, the food ingredient that contains trans fat.
- Include wholesome sources of carbohydrates—fresh fruits and vegetables, whole grains and grain products, legumes, and low-fat dairy products.
- Select foods from all the food groups that provide you with eating satisfaction.
- Find the balance of foods that works best for you. You may prefer to eat slightly larger portions of protein foods like meat and poultry and slightly smaller portions of carbohydrate foods, or you may thrive on larger portions of fiber-rich carbohydrate foods and smaller portions of protein foods. It is a matter of finding what works best for *you*.

# Chapter 6

# Do my genes or metabolism keep me from achieving sustainable weight loss?

Losing weight and sustaining weight loss are not the same for everyone. Each of us is unique. We are born with our own genetic makeup, we make life choices (for example, to smoke, to have children), and we develop a personal biology that affects our ability to achieve lasting weight loss. Although there are individual factors that make weight loss more or less of a challenge, each can be overcome with knowledge and the right tools.

# Myth 6 You can't lose weight if you have the wrong metabolism or genes

*Believers Beware!*

Some people can lose weight and keep it off, but others simply cannot. For them it is not even a remote possibility. There are many factors working against weight loss, so for many people long-term weight management is an unrealistic dream. Some folks are just big-boned, and big-boned people are destined to be big.

Some have the wrong body shape for thinness—naturally big hips and thighs, a round stomach, or overly broad shoulders. Those with slow metabolisms just don't burn a lot of calories. It's especially frustrating for those people because they exercise and don't eat a lot, maybe just a few hundred calories per day, but they can't overcome their body's slow engine.

Some people are born with fat genes. Their mom and dad are big, their grandparents are big, and their cousins are big. The people who come from "big" families have no choice about being big too. Then there are those life events that cause weight gain that can't be reversed: stopping smoking, being pregnant, especially with a second or third child, and menopause. It's impossible for women to combat the natural body changes that come with being female. The weight just piles on even though they're not doing anything differently.

Just as there are people destined to be overweight, there are others who are naturally thin. If they gain a few pounds, they take them right off. Pounds just melt away as soon as they start eating less and exercising more. They are the lucky people.

The unlucky ones cannot lose weight.

## Kernels of Truth

Metabolism affects the rate of weight loss, and people do have different metabolic rates. One way to lose weight is to increase metabolism, to rev up the body's engine so that it burns more calories. Physical activity pumps up the body's metabolism by causing it to work harder during exercise. Building muscle also increases metabolism. Any way to speed up metabolism will burn more calories.

A medical problem associated with weight gain is hypothyroidism. The thyroid is a small, butterfly-shaped gland located just below your Adam's apple that produces hormones that affect your body's metabolism and energy level. The most common cause of hypothyroidism is Hashimoto's thyroiditis, a condition where the body's immune system mistakenly attacks the thyroid gland. With hypothyroidism, the thyroid produces too little thyroid hormone, metabolism slows down, and body weight increases. Diagnosis of hypothyroidism is done primarily by measuring serum TSH (thyroid-stimulating hormone) in the blood. The blood tests performed as part of a routine physical examination usually include this test. Treatment of hypothyroidism consists of taking thyroid hormone in pill form on a daily basis. Symptoms of hypothyroidism should clear up within a few months of starting treatment.

Certain circumstances, including genes, race, age, and life cycle status, increase one's vulnerability to weight gain.

- Although the exact numbers vary, some experts say that people with one overweight parent have at least a 40% chance of being overweight.
- In part, genes determine natural body shape and where the body naturally puts on extra fat. Several studies have found that identical twins are likely to share the same body weight tendencies—if one is overweight, chances are that the other one is also.
- Height and weight charts based on the NHANES III surveys in the United States show that overweight and obesity are more

common among non-Hispanic black or Mexican-American women than among non-Hispanic white women.

- Among all men and women in the United States, the prevalence of being overweight or obese goes up as we get older until after age 69.
- Studies show that women often gain more than the recommended amount of weight during pregnancy, then have a hard time taking the weight off after the baby is born. Likewise, the evidence is strong regarding the tendency of women to gain weight during their menopausal years.

## The Whole Truth

### Body Shape

Chapter 2 discussed two different body types. A body shaped like an apple accumulates extra weight around the abdomen. A pear-shaped body adds extra pounds in the hips and thighs. Traditional thinking has been that it is better to be a pear than an apple—people with an apple-shaped body are at greater risk of developing type 2 diabetes, high blood pressure, high blood cholesterol, and heart disease. Body shape, however, does not affect one's ability to lose weight. Apples can lose weight just as quickly or slowly as pears.

### Frame Size

Chapter 2 also explored the background of the old ideal height and weight tables that were based on bone frame size: small frame, medium frame, and large frame. These tables were widely used, even though they were not based on good science.

Many people assumed that because they were large, they had a bone frame size classification that justified weighing more. The chart allowed people with big bones to be heavier than people with small bones. Today, some people believe that body mass index (BMI) does not apply to them because their extra weight is from their big bones or

# Personal Triumph

## Karen Cireddu

OHIO

Karen Cireddu, a customer service representative, could trace her weight gain to several different events. She gained 65 pounds during pregnancy. She began to gain weight after age 30.

"Joining Weight Watchers was meant to be for me. I am off on Wednesday mornings, and I found a Wednesday morning meeting near my home. Although I hide my weight well, I weighed 178 pounds, and that was way too much. I joined Weight Watchers and got off to a great start.

"About two months later, I decided to quit smoking cold turkey. At that time, I was walking 2 miles a day and then having a cigarette. Here I was, trying to lose weight so that I could be healthier and feel good about myself. So I stopped smoking. Weight Watchers helped me quit because it put structure into my life. Also, I get a lot of coaching and encouragement from the meetings."

*"Joining Weight Watchers was meant to be for me."*

Karen lost almost 34 pounds to reach her goal weight and has continued to lose weight.

muscle, not from fat. The truth is that while people do have different frame sizes and it is possible to be overweight on the BMI chart because of extra muscle, most people who weigh too much for their height do so because of excess body fat.

That said, a few studies have been done on the relationship between bone frame size and BMI. What the studies found is that medium and large bone frames are closely related to their percent body fat and BMI—as the bone frame gets bigger, the percent of body fat and BMI both go up. Small bone frames, however, do not have less body fat. This finding helps explain why Asian-Americans, who tend to have smaller bone frames, have a higher disease risk at a lower BMI than people from other ethnic backgrounds. They may have a higher percentage of body fat even though their BMI may be in the normal range.

## Genes

It seems logical that people from "big" families are destined to be overweight. Science has made great strides in understanding the very complicated issue of why some people are more predisposed to gain weight than others. Almost every week we see new studies published about various genetic components of weight gain and obesity.

A few years ago, there was tremendous interest in the discovery of leptin, a hormone thought to be the messenger sent from fat cells to the brain to regulate eating. Rats that did not produce leptin became obese just as people who do not produce insulin get type 1 diabetes. It was argued that people who were overweight or obese somehow had a genetic breakdown in this system and did not produce enough leptin. It was quickly discovered, however, that obese people tend to have higher levels of leptin than those who are thin, and the way leptin works in the body is much more complicated than being a matter of a simple deficiency. In fact, leptin functionality resembles the insulin resistance found in the metabolic syndrome that leads to type 2 diabetes. It seems that when fat cells send leptin through the bloodstream to the brain to tell the brain to stop eating because the body has plenty of fat, the brain somehow does not get the message and the individual keeps eating. It is as though the phone is ringing and no one is answering it!

Leptin seemed like a wonderful answer that might explain a genetic tendency toward obesity. Unfortunately, we now know that the body's regulation of weight and body fat relies on more than just one messenger. It now looks as if there may be twenty, thirty, or even hundreds of different messengers that interact with each other.

This is not to say that genetics do not affect obesity. In fact, obesity researchers believe that there is a strong relationship between a person's genetic makeup and his or her vulnerability to become overweight. But the human genome, or genetic map, changes excruciatingly slowly—probably less than 1% every one hundred thousand years. So how can we explain the fact that obesity rates have soared by 40% in the United States in the last decade? Certainly our genetic makeup has not changed. With the exception of the rare mutations that cause severe morbid obesity, it seems that numerous genes, each with modest effect, contribute to a person's tendency to become overweight. The answer is that we are eating too much and burning off too little.

Many of us do have bodies that are genetically programmed to make us more vulnerable to gaining weight. But biology is not destiny. Weight gain only happens in an environment that leads to eating too much food and getting too little physical activity. For people who find the right balance between food and physical activity to maintain weight loss, having fat genes does not make a difference.

## Pregnancy

The weight gain of pregnancy poses a challenge to many women. Weight is an important medical aspect of pregnancy, so it is carefully monitored as part of prenatal care by an obstetrician. The key to managing weight during the years when you are having children is to follow your doctor's instructions during the pregnancy or pregnancies,

# Personal Triumph

## Michelle Krischke

TEXAS

Michelle Krischke, who has shared her story in several chapters of this book, gained a lot of weight during her pregnancy."

I basically used the excuse that I was pregnant and the baby needed the extra nutrition. So instead of gaining the pound or so per week that doctors recommend, I gained 15 pounds over a two-week period. My doctor was horrified.

"*That strategy of keeping a written record of what I eat is something I still do, close to twenty years later.*"

"After that, I followed his instructions and got my weight back on track. A strategy that worked for me at that time was to write down everything that went into my mouth. That strategy of keeping a written record of what I eat is something I still do, close to twenty years later. I find that it keeps me honest."

then get back to your prepregnancy weight after each delivery. Women who gain excess weight during pregnancy and fail to it afterward are more likely to develop obesity later on.

With an obstetrician's approval, including a program of moderate-intensity physical activity during pregnancy is generally recommended. After giving birth, breast-feeding and exercise may be beneficial to control weight. A structured weight-loss program may also help. In a study that compared a structured weight-loss program that included a sensible approach to eating and exercise with a do-it-yourself approach in the year following pregnancy, the women who participated in the structured program lost over 15 pounds and 6% of their body fat. The women who tried to lose the weight on their own lost nothing. The researchers concluded that women who were overweight going into the pregnancy were unlikely to lose the weight that they gained during the pregnancy without the help of a structured program.

## Menopause

Menopause marks a major life transition for women. A woman's body stops producing estrogen and the body's entire hormone balance changes. During the years immediately before and after menopause, many women experience mood changes, fatigue, and a general lack of energy or motivation. Women also tend to gain weight and, regardless of weight gain, notice a change in their body shape toward a thicker waist and a more apple-shaped body resulting from the lack of estrogen.

The hormone changes that go along with menopause are linked to a type of overweight called android obesity—the accumulation of fat at the waistline. This explains why many menopausal women complain that they are losing their waist seemingly without eating or exercising any differently. One group of researchers, however, found that reduced physical activity but not increased food intake appears to be a predictor of weight gain during the menopause years. It could be that because menopausal women may feel less energetic, they don't put as much effort into their physical activity.

The best advice is to be prepared for these changes with an action plan for avoiding weight gain or regain. The weight gain and increased waist circumference that are associated with menopause can be prevented with long-term lifestyle changes that include diet and physical activity. A study conducted at the University of Pittsburgh found that premenopausal women who reduced their caloric intake by about 1,000 to 1,500 calories per week and increased their physical activity did not gain weight and even reduced their waist circumference in the years around menopause.

## Quitting Smoking

People who stop smoking gain weight. The average weight gain is between 4.5 and 7 pounds, but a small percentage of former smokers gain 28 pounds or more! The good news is that for the average woman the weight gain is temporary. In a study that followed a group of women who quit smoking, the increase in caloric intake and weight gain was temporary, and they returned to their former weight after one year.

Going from being a smoker to being a nonsmoker does have an effect on metabolism, slowing it down by about 100 calories per day with smoking cessation, but that is not enough to account for all the weight gain. The rest comes from eating more, moving around less, or a combination of the two.

Fear of weight gain should not prevent a person from stopping smoking. The health risks of smoking—the increased risk of heart disease and cancer, impaired glucose tolerance, the increased risk of high blood pressure, and numerous other health problems—are far greater than the health risks of a small short-term weight gain when smoking is stopped.

One way to help prevent weight gain is to increase physical activity. Another is to use a nicotine replacement, in particular nicotine gum, to help delay weight gain. In a group of women who had not tried to quit smoking because they were afraid of gaining weight, a diet plus a nicotine gum regimen increased the success rate for smoking cessation and prevented weight gain.

# Personal Triumph

## Shelli Beers

MARYLAND

Shelli Beers, a recreation therapist, was slim until she began college. The freshman 15 became the sophomore 20. Shelli married and divorced shortly afterward and found herself alone and lonely in a town where she knew very few people. Food became her friend, and she gained even more weight.

"One morning, I could not find a pair of jeans in my closet that fit. I had been trying to lose weight by just exercising, but obviously it was not working. So I joined Weight Watchers because a couple of women at work had been successful on the program.

*"I lost 56 pounds to my goal weight. Today, I am the same weight that I was in high school."*

"I lost 56 pounds to my goal weight. Today, I am the same weight that I was in high school. I have maintained my weight, even after having a hysterectomy that forced my body into menopause and not being able to exercise during the recovery from the surgery. Weight Watchers has really worked for me despite the hurdles in my life."

*Have you ever heard...*

**Have you ever heard . . . "Some people can eat all they want and never gain weight."**

Wouldn't you like to be the lucky person who can eat everything and anything and not gain weight? Metabolism in fact does vary from person to person, but the idea that there are some people who can eat all they want and never gain weight simply is not true. Some people regulate themselves by eating a big meal on occasion, followed by very small meals the next day. Others have an extremely active lifestyle that burns a lot of calories through activity and increased metabolism. Don't be fooled! Most people who eat a lot and do not gain weight work very hard to keep their weight steady whether they talk about it or not.

## Slow Metabolism

It seems as if every discussion about weight somehow turns into a discussion about metabolism. Because the two are closely related, the assumption is often made that if a person is overweight, it follows that the excess weight is due to a slow metabolism. It is true that metabolism tends to slow down as the years go by. But the slowdown is not automatic. Here's why.

The body's organs and, even more so, muscles, drive metabolism. Metabolism has three major components: resting metabolic rate, metabolism of activity, and energy spent digesting and absorbing food. Resting metabolism is the amount of energy the body uses to keep all systems going day in and day out; it is the energy that is burned by the brain, heart, kidneys, and all the organs and cells in the body. About two-thirds to three-quarters of the energy we burn every day goes into the simple process of keeping the body alive. The second major component of metabolism is the energy that we burn in activities such as walking, stair climbing, picking up children, and participating in planned physical activity. Finally, a relatively small percentage of calories are burned in the process of digesting and absorbing food. These components add up to our total metabolism. Metabolism is measured in calories.

Each year, metabolism tends to slow a bit because most people inadvertently reduce their physical activity. This decrease in activity delivers a double whammy to metabolism. The body burns fewer calories because it spends less time doing physical activity. Slowly, almost imperceptibly, it also loses lean muscle tissue because the muscles are less active, a true case of use it or lose it.

The average adult over age 20 loses half a pound of lean muscle tissue every year. Why is this important? If you are 30 years old and have lost 5 pounds of lean muscle tissue over the past decade, your resting metabolism is burning fewer calories simply to fuel basic needs. Your metabolism has in fact slowed down.

Keep in mind that weight loss affects metabolism because a smaller body has less lean muscle tissue. The metabolism of a person who was overweight and has lost weight is the same as the metabolism of a person who was never overweight in the first place. With less mass to move around, the body spends fewer calories.

We learned earlier in this chapter that non-Hispanic black women tend to have higher BMIs than white non-Hispanic women. One reason may be metabolism. African-American women tend to have lower resting metabolic rates. This does not mean that sustained weight loss is not possible for African-American women. Rather, it means that their rate of weight loss is likely to be a bit slower and that the daily caloric intake needed to sustain the loss will be a bit lower.

## Thinking Does Not Equal Doing

By some accounts, the typical American underestimates caloric intake by 400 to 500 calories per day. Women tend to underestimate their caloric intake by 20%. A woman who is working on weight loss and thinks that she is following a 1,200-calorie diet is actually more likely to be eating about 1,450 calories per day. Part of the error is in portion size—thinking that a portion size is smaller than it really is. The other problem is that people remember eating healthier foods and forget about the less healthy ones. This is particularly true of snack foods, like a small candy bar or a handful of chips, perhaps because these foods are often eaten as a quick snack and not part of a regular meal. For example, a person is likely to remember eating a bowl of cereal, banana, and skim milk at breakfast but to underestimate the size of the cheeseburger that was eaten for lunch or forget the few french fries taken from a coworker's plate at the same lunch.

A classic study looked at "weight-loss-resistant" women who consistently indicated that they ate less than 1,200 calories per day but were not able to lose weight. The researchers found that the women were not losing weight because they were eating more calories than they thought. Their metabolism was fine.

This study has been replicated many times over, each time with the same results. The women were not lying; they truly believed that they were eating less. For this reason, recalling or tracking food intake is an unreliable method for determining whether a person has a slow metabolism.

Any suspected metabolic cause for weight gain or the inability to lose weight should be checked through medically reliable testing. This testing should extend beyond the usual thyroid function studies or keeping food records to include resting metabolic rate.

Just as people tend to underestimate how much they eat, they tend to overestimate their physical activity. Keep in mind, as shown in chapter 4, that it takes a lot of physical activity to make a difference in calorie burning. People also are somewhat misled by the calorie counts provided by exercise machines. Exercise machines tend to overestimate the actual number of calories burned in a session by as much as 30%; machines that request information on the user's weight tend to be more accurate.

## The Bottom Line

Biology is not destiny. Many different factors affect weight loss to a mild degree, but no one factor prevents weight loss. It is true that some people have a genetic or a personal profile that makes them more vulnerable to weight gain. Nonetheless, it is possible to prevent the weight gain from happening and to lose weight if it has already been gained. Sustained weight loss is possible for virtually anyone.

## Weight Loss That Lasts

# Action Steps

Knowledge is power. Understanding your personal circumstances and how they may affect both your metabolism and your weight loss helps to develop approaches and strategies that will work for you.

- Take a look at your individual circumstances and set realistic weight-loss goals based on what you see. For example, if you have recently quit smoking or come from a family with weight issues, a weekly weight loss of ½ to 1 pound may be a better target than 1½ to 2 pounds.
- If you are genetically vulnerable to gaining weight, be particularly diligent about creating a daily eating plan and schedule for physical activity. If you have children and are concerned about their having inherited your genetic tendencies, be sure to be a good role model for them and show them that successful weight management is possible because you are doing it.
- Stay physically active as a way to minimize your body's loss of lean muscle tissue. Once you are at your weight goal, you may even reverse the process and start to increase the amount of lean muscle tissue in your body.
- Keep a positive mindset. Despite your individual circumstances, you can lose weight and keep it off!

# Chapter 7

# Is my metabolism affected by what, how, and when I eat?

Whenever the talk turns to the science of weight loss, you hear the word *metabolism* a lot. It is often thought of as the Holy Grail of weight loss. Find a way to boost metabolism and the pounds will fall off. And if it is possible to speed up the metabolism without making any changes in how you live your life, so much the better!

It is easy to believe the pseudoscience that talks up ways to boost metabolism to lose weight. This chapter explores the realities behind foods, food combinations, meal timing, and other factors that may or may not speed up metabolism and contribute to weight loss.

# Myth 7

## You can boost your metabolism by what, how, and when you eat

*Believers Beware!*

Weight loss is about burning more calories than you eat. The traditional way to lose weight is to eat less and exercise more. But the secret of *superior* weight loss is to speed up metabolism so that weight is lost automatically. After all, it is the body's metabolism that sets the pace for burning calories.

Rather than accept a slow metabolism, it makes more sense to make the one you have go faster. There are lots of magazine articles and television programs explaining that what and how we eat and exercise affects our metabolism. The good news is that you can boost your metabolism with virtually no effort. So it makes sense that making some minor changes in those areas can create a metabolic advantage that speeds weight loss. There are so many choices—exercises, special foods and food combinations, and dozens of other things—all designed to raise the body's metabolism. Going this route makes weight loss faster and easier.

## Kernels of Truth

Since the beginning of time, people have expanded the powers of food beyond simply meeting nutritional and energy needs. The belief that specific foods can cure health problems is a longstanding cultural tradition: eating chicken soup to cure a cold and oysters to enhance fertility are just two examples. We really want to believe in the power of foods. It is not surprising that specific foods and eating regimens have made their way into the folklore of weight loss. With great optimism, people embrace the latest new food or way of eating with the hope that it will put them on the path to sustained weight loss.

The magic of a single solution for weight loss focuses on just one aspect of a food, supplement, or activity. This is similar to the tale about the three blind men and the elephant: Three blind men are asked to describe an elephant. One of them touches the trunk, another touches the tail, and the third touches the foot. Each of the blind men accurately describes what he touched, but none of them can describe the elephant because the animal is bigger than a single body part.

Weight-loss myths are similar in that they isolate a particular feature that may be true and offer it as a solution to the entire problem of weight loss. It is possible to find at least one study to prove that each of the weight-loss boosters below does lead to superior weight loss. Often the one study that is publicized on television or read about in a magazine is the only study that shows results, but it is easy to believe the story because the study results are true, even if only just once.

But rigorous science requires a study to be replicated by other scientists and for them to observe the same results. Few of us have the inclination to track down all the research studies on a topic in order to find out if there is general agreement about the pool of scientific evidence on a specific weight-loss booster. We have done so for you. When the scientific community makes its judgment on a particular issue, it is based on all of the evidence, not just on one or a few isolated studies.

Building more muscle mass does increase metabolism. Because

**Highly Touted Weight-Loss Boosters**

- Aerobics that burn calories after the exercise is done
- Weight lifting
- Weight-loss dietary supplements
- High-protein diet
- Eating more frequently
- Not eating after 7:00 P.M.
- Avoiding certain food combinations
- Eating hot peppers with every meal
- Eating only fruit in the morning

muscle is the engine that drives the body, it burns more calories than fat, so activities that speed up metabolism can boost calorie burning and weight loss.

Is it possible to lose weight on diets that promise to speed up metabolism? Probably not. If you do lose weight, it is not due to a faster metabolism. Read on to discover that the secret to weight loss is calories and that the weight loss achieved through a metabolism-boosting diet is also due to calories.

## The Whole Truth

### It's All about Calories

Body weight reflects the balance between calories in and calories out. As described in the previous chapter, the food we eat supplies calories. Our body burns calories three ways: through resting metabolism, the calories burned as the body keeps itself running 24/7; during physical activity; and in digesting and absorbing food. A steady body weight means a balance between food and calorie burning. Gaining or losing weight is the sign of an imbalance.

# *Personal Triumph*

## Sherry Dieckman

ILLINOIS

Sherry Dieckman is a retired schoolteacher who struggled with her weight throughout childhood and most of her adult life. When Sherry joined Weight Watchers, she weighed close to 200 pounds.

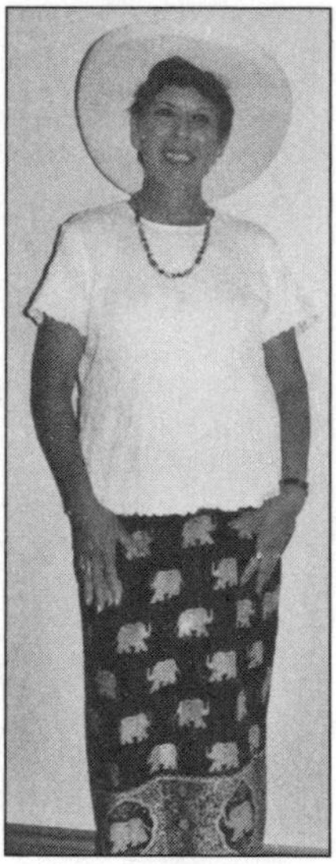

"In the past, the only thing that had helped me lose weight was diet pills. None of the other approaches I tried worked for very long because they didn't fit my lifestyle. Eventually, my doctor suggested gastric bypass surgery, which I really didn't want. So I joined Weight Watchers.

"What I learned at Weight Watchers was that I could adjust my eating to fit my lifestyle. Here is the magic—the weight started coming off and I felt like I wasn't doing anything special or different. For example, I happen to have a sweet tooth and I will not give up sweets! Here is what I do—I exercise for an hour every evening, and then I enjoy dessert. The beauty of Weight Watchers is that you can make the program work for you no matter what type of person you are. This is a lifestyle change, not a diet. Every time I buy kitty litter, I remind myself of how much weight I lost—over two 25-pound bags of kitty litter!"

*"Because my husband and I were so successful at losing weight, our son and daughter-in-law joined also."*

**Calories and Weight**

| | |
|---|---|
| Calories in greater than calories out | Weight gain |
| Calories in equal to calories out | Steady weight |
| Calories in less than calories out | Weight loss |

The *only* scientifically proven method for losing weight involves the creation of a caloric imbalance. At the end of the day, the only true way to lose weight is to eat fewer calories in food and/or burn more calories. This has been shown time and time again in decades of rigorous scientific studies. One example of the hundreds that exist was done in Switzerland. Fifty-four obese people had their calories restricted to 1,100 per day. Different combinations of foods and meal timing were tested. There was no difference in weight losses; only the calories made a difference.

## A Faster Metabolism Burns More

It takes a shortfall of about 500 calories a day to lose 1 pound per week and 1,000 calories a day to lose 2 pounds weekly. The most effective method to create this shortfall is to cut calories from food and also to boost metabolism. But despite the promises of so many popular diets and products, metabolism can be boosted in only a couple of ways: exercising more and speeding up heart rate.

One of the chief benefits of exercise is that it revs up metabolism. The reason is simple. Individuals who exercise on a consistent basis maintain high levels of lean muscle tissue throughout their lifetime. They also build new muscle. Lean muscle tissue sustains high levels of metabolism. In fact, lean muscle tissue burns seventy times as many calories as fat does. Exercise burns calories, and longer periods of exercise mean greater calorie burning.

While it is true that an increase in lean muscle mass increases metabolism because muscles burn a lot of calories, weight loss almost always results in some loss of muscle mass. The muscles have less weight to carry around, so less muscle is needed. People who follow extreme diets to get a fast weight loss can significantly reduce their lean muscle tissue and thereby slow their metabolism.

A popular theory widely reported in the media is that exercise increases metabolism during activity and for a period of time after the activity is completed. Unfortunately, studies that have researched this concept do not have consistent results. In general, studies on humans suggest that metabolism increases when the amount of body muscle increases but that the number of extra calories burned after exercise is relatively small. And no studies have directly linked the aftereffects of exercise with significant weight loss. It's the calories expended doing the exercise that boost weight loss, not the aftereffects of exercise on metabolism.

The second way to increase metabolism is to increase heart rate. The heart and other organs contribute to the resting metabolic rate—the calories the body burns just to keep itself going. In a controlled study that looked at the effects of amphetamines on weight loss, the stimulants caused greater weight loss. Heart rate and blood pressure went up and food intake went down, a side effect of feeling hyper and too nervous to eat. Many weight-loss supplements contain chemical or herbal stimulants, including caffeine, guarana, and the now-banned ephedra, which speed up metabolism by pumping up the heart rate. Most of the supplements and over-the-counter products that are marketed to promote weight loss contain stimulants, albeit at a lesser strength than that found in prescription amphetamines. Like their more potent cousin, these compounds are marketed as "fat-burning" and cause weight loss by increasing your heart rate and blood pressure and decreasing your appetite.

These stimulants can work, but they do so at a cost to the body. Negative side effects include insomnia, nervousness, anxiety, and in extreme cases, death. Increasingly, some of these products (including the ones that were most effective, like phenylpropanolamine and ephedra) have been banned because of the negative side effects.

A careful look at the ingredient list of many herbal remedies reveals the truth—herbal diuretics that cause the body to lose fluid through urination and herbal laxatives. Just because the package says the product is natural or herbal does not mean it is healthy. A combination of stimulants, diuretics, and laxatives does not add up to a safe and sensible way to lose weight.

Over the years, other foods and products have been falsely promoted as metabolism boosters for weight loss. Grapefruit, for example, was said to have compounds that speed up metabolism; an added promise was that eating and digesting grapefruit actually uses up more calories than are in the grapefruit. Celery is often promoted as a food that burns more calories than it supplies. But there is no scientific proof that calories spent digesting and absorbing can be pumped up by eating particular foods.

*Have you ever heard . . .*

**"There are weight-loss vitamins that boost metabolism."**

There are several brands of "weight-conscious" vitamin-mineral supplements available today. While they vary in their ingredients, many contain herbs or extracts that speed up the heart rate and therefore the metabolism. Many make claims that they contain added amounts of the vitamins (for example, B vitamins) or minerals (for example, chromium) that are essential to process energy within the body. Although the statements are true, there are no rigorous scientific trials demonstrating that taking these supplements improves weight-loss success.

### The Source of Calories Does Not Affect Your Weight Loss

Which is best for weight loss—a diet low in carbohydrates and high in protein, or a diet balanced in carbohydrates, protein, and fat? That's been a question that has received a lot of scientific attention, and science is showing a firm conclusion—it does not matter. According to dozens of research studies, no particular type of diet speeds up metabolism more than another. In 2004, a complete review of all research studies on the topic concluded that following a low-carbohydrate and/or high-protein diet did not affect the rate of metabolism. Diets with differing proportions of macronutrients work because they reduce calories, albeit in disguise. They have no special effects on metabolism.

### Eat More, Lose Weight?

Diets that promise more food for greater weight loss are usually variations on very low-fat diets. Because they focus on naturally low-fat, low-calorie foods like fruits and vegetables, they supply a greater volume of food for fewer calories. The foods are also ones that are thought of as harder to digest, suggesting that they burn more calories during digestion. However, as with other types of diets, very low-fat diets work because they are lower in calories. They do not speed up metabolism and do not require digestion to go into overdrive.

### No Food or Food Combination Burns Body Fat

The term *thermogenesis*, or calorie burning, became very popular in the mid-1990s when a popular weight-loss book suggested that certain foods caused the body to burn extra energy in order to digest and absorb them. The concept of thermogenesis is based on science, but the relative contribution of this extra energy burning is so minor that it is irrelevant for weight loss.

"Fat-burning" foods do not burn fat. Highly acidic foods like grapefruit, lemon juice, and vinegar are said to melt away fat because they are so acidic. This explanation sounds logical but does not work in real life. Certain food combinations are said to create chemical reactions in the body that promote loss of body fat. This promise cannot be proven, and these foods do not boost metabolism.

Some foods like caffeine-containing beverages and capsaicin-containing chile peppers have been linked with a boost in calorie burning. Caffeine is a mild stimulant, and high dosages of caffeine raise the heart rate. Chile peppers cause the body to sweat and to feel stimulated. In one study, capsaicin did cause increased fat burning in a group of people who had lost weight, but it did not help them maintain their weight loss. Results were similar for green tea, a beverage that contains caffeine and other components reported to boost metabolism. When put into rigorous studies, neither demonstrated a significant effect on weight loss.

## Eating Patterns Do Not Make a Difference

Eating three times daily or six times daily? Having a small breakfast and big dinner or big breakfast and small dinner? Which is best for burning calories? Again, it does not matter. *As long as calories remain the same,* meal sizes relative to each other do not affect weight loss. A series of well-controlled experiments that looked at the effect of meal timing on metabolism was conducted in a clinical research center at a university. Regardless of the meal timing—eating once a day or several times a day, eating at night or in the morning—weight loss stayed the same when study subjects ate the same number of calories. The researchers concluded that the body's regulatory systems are extremely fine-tuned.

So if meal timing does not change metabolism, how does meal timing work? It promotes weight loss by throwing off normal eating routines in a way that leads to eating fewer calories. Say that you are told to eat only fruit before noon. If you are a breakfast eater, then not being able to eat cereal, toast, a sausage biscuit, or your usual breakfast foods automatically cuts calories. There is nothing metabolically magical about eating only fruit in the morning. The same is true if you tend to snack in the evening and go on a "metabolism-boosting" diet that prohibits eating after 7:00 P.M.

That said, meal timing is important because eating plans have to be livable and adaptable to our different lifestyles. Work schedule, family structure, exercise routine, and numerous other factors help determine the best eating schedule. Say a person works the night shift and sleeps during the day. She may want to eat dinner with her family even though that meal is really breakfast for her, then eat lunch in the middle of her work shift and a small breakfast with her family before going to sleep. A person who works full-time and exercises daily after work may want to eat breakfast, lunch, then two mini-meals, one midafternoon before exercise and one at night after exercise. No one schedule is better than another.

You may have heard how important it is to eat breakfast. It is true that numerous studies have shown that people who eat breakfast are much less likely to gain weight than those who do not eat breakfast. Eating breakfast provides essential nutrients, sets the body up with energy for the day, and is linked with less eating later in the day. The effect is not on metabolism; it is on lifestyle and habits.

Some weight-loss proponents recommend eating a bigger breakfast, followed by a smaller lunch and an even smaller dinner. The theory is that the majority of calories are eaten toward the beginning of the day when the body needs them most. This approach works in theory but has not undergone the rigorous studies needed to prove or disprove its impact on sustained weight loss. It is also not practical for most people.

## Restrictive Diets Reduce Calories

As with diets that throw off eating routines by changing meal timing, a diet that imposes almost any type of restriction will reduce calories by forcing a change in habits. Whether it's avoiding gluten and dairy, not eating a protein food and a starch within four hours of each other, consuming bowls of cabbage soup, or only eating fruit before noon, following rules that restrict the type of food eaten, the time of day food is eaten, or how frequently a food or food type is eaten will reduce caloric intake.

Let's look more closely at the concept of separating different types of foods. Say that a diet is based on avoiding eating starches and protein foods together in a meal, a basic premise of a popular diet in the 1990s. That means no cereal (starch) and milk (protein) or toast (starch) and egg (protein) at breakfast, no sandwich at lunch because starchy bread typically is combined with a protein food, and no potato, rice, pasta, or bread (all starches) with meat, chicken, or fish (all proteins) at dinner. Imagine how much less you would eat if you were told to avoid traditional food combinations!

What about eating three standard-size meals and no snacks versus eating six or even eight mini-meals? The end result depends on the routine that is being changed and the total amount of food eaten. A frequent snacker might eat less food on a three-meal no-snack diet and lose weight. The mini-meal eater could lose weight as long as the calories in the mini-meals added up to less than he or she was eating before. The science in this area is inconsistent. Some research says that eating fewer, bigger meals allows the body to burn a few more calories digesting and absorbing foods. But there is no strong research showing that meal frequency and size affects weight loss as long as calories are the same.

### The Placebo Effect Works

For every one of the myths and gimmicks about foods, supplements, and food timing and combining discussed in this chapter, there are a dozen more being promoted. These myths are so prevalent because each has a kernel of truth—a small part of the myth based on science. It is the fantastic story that gets wrapped up with the truth that creates a myth rather than a valid, long-lasting way to lose weight.

The placebo effect happens when a person believes that there is a direct cause-and-effect relationship between two things even if it does not exist. Because the person believes in the relationship, however, his or her behavior changes in a way that produces the anticipated effect.

Rigorous scientific studies include a placebo group and a group that is actually getting the treatment. This is the only valid way to ensure that it is the treatment and not the placebo that is producing the effect. Many promising treatments in the area of weight loss lose their luster when they are evaluated in a rigorous scientific study that includes a placebo group. For example, acupuncture is often touted as a weight-loss treatment. When tested against a placebo, however, it has been shown to be ineffective. The same has been shown for subliminal tapes to induce weight loss.

## It's about Behavior Change, Not Metabolism

Ultimately, behavior changes that support eating fewer calories and being more active lead to weight loss. Despite this reality, only one-third of Americans trying to lose weight use the strategy that is the

# Personal Triumph

## Jerry McNeight

OREGON

Jerry McNeight, a trucking analyst, gained weight after undergoing knee and hip replacements to treat damage done by years of mountain climbing and extreme sports. Jerry tried many different weight-loss approaches before joining Weight Watchers.

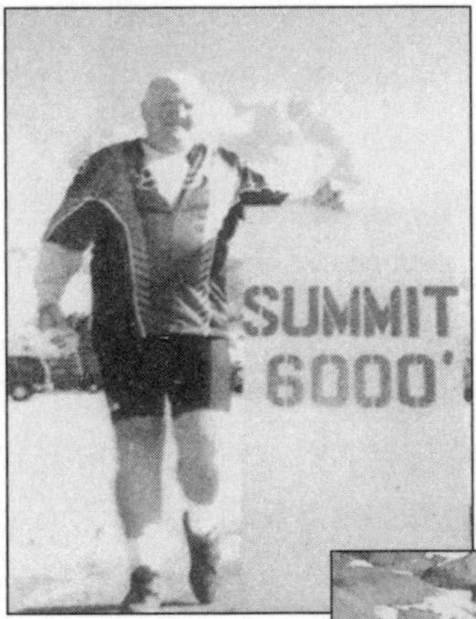


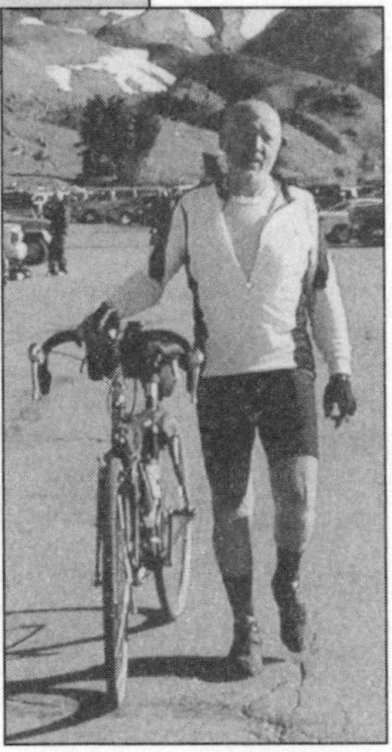

"I tried pills that promised weight loss while I slept. That was a joke. I cut my carbohydrates once and lost lots of weight—but then I gained back all the weight.

*"What I like about Weight Watchers is that it is very practical."*

"What I like about Weight Watchers is that it is very practical. I don't have to eat special foods or live on one particular type of food. It's all about eating sensible amounts and being physically active."

fundamental foundation of weight loss. Sustainable weight loss does not result from a revved-up metabolism or the unique properties of specific foods. However, particular eating behaviors and patterns, such as meal frequency, meal timing, or following a specific dietary pattern, and nutritional factors, like the energy density of food and the amount of fiber, may affect caloric intake and thus weight loss.

Here is an example of a suggested behavior change that works, even though the premise for the change has nothing to do with a metabolism. Many programs will tell you that you should not eat after 7:00 P.M. because "food eaten in the evening turns to fat." The truth is that any food turns to fat if calories in are greater than calories out. The time of day that it is eaten does not matter. However, many people consume a large portion of their daily calories in the evening. Television viewing, an evening activity for many, is also associated with increased caloric intake and "mindless" snacking. A dietary regimen that restricts evening eating works because it limits calories. That, in turn, helps burn fat.

## The Bottom Line

The famous baby doctor Benjamin Spock was known for telling young mothers, "Trust yourself, you know more than you think you do." The same holds true for weight loss. There is no reason to feel bad if you have tried the diets and products that promise a metabolism-inspired weight loss. Everybody wants to believe in the promise, and the pseudoscience that goes along with many of the claims seems to make a lot of sense. But when it comes to achieving weight loss that lasts, a combination of instinct and a complete disclosure of the pool of scientific studies is the way to figure out what is real and what is a myth.

It is much more important to find an eating style and exercise routine that suits your life and that you can stay with over time than trying to follow an uncomfortable or overly restricted regimen in the hopes of boosting your metabolism. Ultimately, it is livable changes to your lifestyle that will make the big difference and help you lose the weight and keep it off.

## Weight Loss That Lasts

# Action Steps

Armed with good scientific knowledge, you can evaluate if and how a weight-loss product or method will lead to weight loss. It is important to take the time to research and analyze any weight-loss approach before using it to safeguard your health and bank account.

- Ask yourself the following questions the next time that you hear about a new approach to weight loss:
  - Does it promise to help the body burn more calories? How?
  - How does it propose to increase your metabolism? Is this valid based on what you now know?
  - Does it increase your lean body mass to help your body burn more calories?
  - Does it increase your heart rate?
  - Does it help you consume fewer calories than you are burning?
- Do a little informal research when you hear about new weight-loss theories. The Internet can be a terrific resource for information as long as you stick to reliable sources. Seek out credible sources like the National Institutes of Health Weight Control Information Network (www.niddk.nih.gov/health/nutrit/win.htm), the American Obesity Association (www.obesity.org), the American Dietetic Association (www.eatright.org), Tufts University Nutrition Navigator (www.navigator.tufts.edu), and Weight Watchers (www.WeightWatchers.com).
- Find the eating pattern that is satisfying for you and that fits your lifestyle. You may prefer eating just three meals daily, three meals plus a snack, or more frequent, smaller meals. By all means experiment until you find the balance between satisfying your hunger, fitting food into your lifestyle, and regulating what and how much you eat.

# Chapter 8

# Does how I lose weight really matter?

It may sound sensible to capitalize on the deep motivation you are feeling today and to make drastic changes to get your excess pounds off as quickly as possible. You might be considering methods that lead you to lose weight faster than others. In fact, the more extreme the method (that is, the severity of the food or exercise changes required), the faster the weight will come off. This chapter examines the facts and fallacies of the "I'll do whatever it takes to get the weight off fast" syndrome of weight loss.

# Myth 8 It doesn't matter how you take the weight off; you can think about keeping it off later

*Believers Beware!*

Weight loss is a war and those extra pounds are the enemy. The best way to lose weight is with a warrior's attitude—attack it with a vengeance. Reaching your weight-loss goal means total victory . . . and the end of the war.

It's okay—in fact, it is necessary—to make big sacrifices in order to win the weight war. After all, too much indulgence caused the weight gain, so what's a little bit of punishment to get rid of it? The faster and harsher the punishment, the sooner the war is won and it's possible to return to normal. How the weight is lost doesn't matter—if it's with a diet or method that's extreme, that's okay because it will be over that much sooner.

Sure, doctors say that quick weight loss is bad for health, but so what? Once the weight is off, the long-term benefits more than make up for any short-term damage. Better looks, a new wardrobe, and greater happiness—it's all worth it.

And who needs to worry right now about keeping the weight off? That can be dealt with later. After all, it's impossible to focus on more than one thing at a time, and right now the focus needs to be 150% on getting the weight off.

## Kernels of Truth

Weight gain is not associated with positive thoughts, so it is not surprising that a person who decides to lose weight often approaches it with a take-no-prisoners attitude. The intense motivation, dedication, and optimism that often initiate a weight-loss effort are terrific! And getting some good results early in the process is important. The Institute of Medicine (IOM) notes that a good weight loss in the first days and weeks of a weight-loss attempt is predictive of overall success.

All of us like to be rewarded for our efforts. That's why losing weight quickly can be so satisfying. The feedback is virtually instantaneous—the number on the scale goes down daily, sometimes by even a full pound.

Any regimen that restricts food intake will lead to weight loss as long as you are eating fewer calories than you burn. It doesn't matter whether the calories are cut by eliminating a major food group, cutting out certain foods, eating less of everything, or replacing meals with drinks, bars, or packaged foods.

Weight loss brings big health benefits. Several studies have shown that losing weight leads to decreases in disease risk factors like total and LDL ("bad") cholesterol, blood pressure, and blood sugar. It does not take long for these risk factors to go down. Changes can be measured in a matter of days or weeks.

While losing weight and sustaining weight loss are often thought of as separate events, they are very much related. The first chapter of this book includes a list of success factors for losing weight and a slightly different list for keeping the weight off. Taken together, the lists are more similar than not, and the factors that predict sustained weight loss are extensions of the same factors needed for successful weight loss.

# *Personal Triumph*

## Rebecca Hill

CALIFORNIA

Rebecca Hill is a television postproduction coordinator who gained weight from the stress of work. Rebecca had a stubborn 15 to 30 pounds that she had taken off and regained constantly since college.

"I now realize that I was thinking only about getting the weight off as fast as possible. I would diet as a quick fix in order to fit into a certain dress or prepare for an upcoming beauty pageant. I was either dieting to get ready for a pageant or gorging myself afterward on blueberry pancakes, fried chicken, mashed potatoes, and everything else that had been off limits to me.

> *"Nothing is off limits; I simply have to make good decisions one day at a time."*

"What I learned when I joined Weight Watchers was that losing weight meant changing my lifestyle. I used to avoid certain foods; now I don't because sustaining my weight loss is a lifestyle I will be living with forever. Nothing is off limits; I simply have to make good decisions one day at a time. For instance, if I know I'm going to eat pizza for lunch, I make sure I eat a lighter breakfast and plan for a lighter dinner."

Rebecca reached her goal weight loss of over 41 pounds.

# The Whole Truth

## The Method Matters

In the war against excess pounds, true victory is weight loss that lasts. To claim victory in your battle of the bulge, you need to think like a general, choosing strategies and tactics that will lead you to your goal weight and then keep you there. More than anything else, the method by which you lose weight determines how successful you will be.

While the temptation may be great to choose the method you believe will take the weight off fastest, it can also be a mistake. Most weight-loss methods will include some kind of eating and activity component. But how the method requires you put these components into practice needs to be evaluated to see if you are taking careless health risks, if you may be setting yourself up for out-of-control eating, or if the composition of the pounds you are losing is helping or hurting your weight-loss efforts. While the goal of weight loss is to lose the fat, depending on the weight-loss method you choose, the pounds you lose may be more water and muscle than fat. Choosing a comprehensive weight-loss method will help you lose fat, tone your body and muscles, and build skills that will help you keep the weight off.

## Early Weight Loss Is More Water Than Fat

Virtually any weight-loss method produces a rapid drop in pounds during the first few days and weeks. This phenomenon is a natural part of the weight-loss process and reinforces the decision to lose weight in the first place. However, the pounds that are lost in the early days need to be kept in perspective. The purpose of losing weight is to lose body fat. And while it would be wonderful if all of the pounds lost early were fat, that is not the case.

A person needs to accumulate a caloric deficit of about 3,500 calories to lose a single pound of fat. To lose 5 pounds in one week, one would have to eliminate 17,500 calories, or 2,500 calories per day. Most people do not even eat 2,500 calories daily. If the weight loss is not fat, what is it? Numerous studies have looked into this and they always come back with the same answer: the early weight loss most diets bring is mostly water.

The human body, with all its component parts of blood, bone, muscle, and fat, is made up largely of water. Fat-free mass is 70% to 75% water, and body fat is 10% to 40% water. The more fat a body carries, the lower the water content of the fat. For the average adult woman, 50% of her body weight is water; for the average adult man, 59% of his body weight is water. Women have less body water than men because they are less muscular, so they have a smaller fat-free mass. Regardless of gender, however, water is part of every single cell in the human body.

Let's take a brief look at why the body sheds water in the early days of weight loss. Glycogen is a type of carbohydrate that the body stores in the liver and muscle. It is like a sponge, holding on to three or four times its weight in water. During the early days of weight loss, the body releases and burns its glycogen for extra energy since food calories have been reduced. As the glycogen is burned, it lets go of its water. The result is that the body loses a total of 4 or 5 grams of weight for every gram of glycogen that is burned.

The next time you are at the market, pick up a bottle of water. You will quickly notice that water is heavy—a pint weighs 1 pound; a gallon weighs 8 pounds. When you lose body water with early weight loss, you notice the pounds on the scale. This creates the illusion that a great deal of weight is being lost. A lot of weight *is* being lost because water is so heavy. But this is not sustainable weight loss because the body eventually gains back the lost water. We all need a certain level of body fluid in order for our bodies to function properly.

Once the body uses up its glycogen, it begins to burn fat for energy. Each gram of fat has more than twice the calories of a gram of glycogen. That means you need to burn more than double the calories to lose 1 gram of fat as you would need to lose 1 gram of glycogen. Fat also does not store much water. Weight loss defined by the pounds on the bathroom scale is much slower when the body burns fat. The natural course of weight loss is a quick loss from water followed by a significant slowdown as the body pulls from fat stores to meet its energy needs.

| BURNING GLYCOGEN VERSUS BURNING FAT | | |
|---|---|---|
| Type of Fuel | Calories per Gram | Weight Lost in Burning 100 Calories |
| Glycogen | 4 | 100–125 grams |
| Fat | 9 | 12–15 grams |

The rate of weight loss after the body uses up its glycogen stores should average 1 to 2 pounds per week. More rapid weight loss is too fast and means that the body is losing excess pounds from one of two places. The first is less common—additional water loss from a health complication like heart failure or a serious gastrointestinal disease. The second source of extra energy for the body is muscle, which is lean tissue or fat-free mass.

## Fast Weight Loss Equals Muscle Loss

One problem with extreme diets is that they often lead to muscle loss. The faster the weight loss, the more likely it is that a significant portion will be lean muscle. Muscle loss works directly against sustained weight loss.

Drastically reducing calories forces the body to rely more and more on lean tissue—muscle—to meet its energy needs. As calories are restricted, the body starts turning to any energy source it can find to fuel its daily energy needs. The body literally starts to cannibalize itself. In many extreme weight-loss methods, as much as 40% of the weight lost may be from lean muscle! Muscle tissue, like glycogen, is about 80% water. So when the body breaks down muscle tissue, weight loss is quicker because of the water that is released.

Why is this problematic? Think of your body as an automobile, with muscle as the engine and fat as the trunk that stores energy. If you cut down on the size of the engine, then the amount of energy that your body burns decreases. This is exactly what happens when you lose lean muscle mass. What a pity it would be to go through all the sacrifice and struggle to reach a lower weight and then end up with a smaller engine that burns fewer calories.

There are two strategies for maintaining lean muscle during weight loss. The first is to pace your weight loss. You can help maintain the size of your engine and lessen the likelihood of regaining pounds if you lose weight at the recommended pace of 1 to 2 pounds per week. Pacing your weight loss means that your diet is supplying enough calories to allow fat burning but prevent muscle loss. Second, regular exercise is important, particularly during weight loss, to preserve lean muscle tissue. Although exercise helps preserve lean tissue, it cannot undo the damage done by too-fast weight loss. An extreme diet that supplies too few calories causes the body to break down muscle even if the person is exercising. In a study that compared a very low-calorie diet with resistance exercise and the same 800-calorie diet without resistance training, the loss of fat-free mass was the same.

### Other Problems with Extreme Methods

Any method that produces fast weight loss by definition needs to be extreme. Severely limiting calories creates nutritional imbalances. Single-food diets (for example, the cabbage soup diet), eliminating

*Have you ever heard . . .*

**"It doesn't matter if an extreme method is unhealthy. There is plenty of time to establish healthier habits once the weight is off."**

There are two problems with this statement. First, it is possible to do significant damage to health even with short-term use of an extreme diet. Second, following an extreme approach to lose weight quickly is a recipe for regaining the weight. It is far better to fine-tune weight management so that initial strategies are consistent with long-term strategies. This way, the positive changes that are made as weight loss progresses become incorporated into the fabric of your life, setting up the framework for sustainable weight loss.

foods with particular macronutrients like carbohydrates or fats, and skipping meals are examples of the extreme methods often used to attain fast weight loss.

Rapid weight loss is associated with a host of health problems including hair loss, dry skin, irritability, and commonly gallstone formation. Extreme methods are a setup for weight-loss failure. They provide fast weight loss for only as long as they are followed. But very few people can stay with them for more than a few days or weeks. Once the method is abandoned, old habits return and so does the weight. Several studies that have evaluated weight regain after completion of a very low-calorie diet have found that unless the lifestyle changes that support long-term weight loss are made, the pounds are quickly regained.

## Extreme Diets and Eating Behavior

Because extreme diets are so difficult to follow, they require maintaining a very high level of dietary restraint. In a study that looked specifically at dietary restraint, researchers found that high levels of dietary restraint and rigid control of eating were associated with higher scores of disinhibition and more frequent, severe episodes of overeating. Dietary restriction for fast weight loss can create a rebound effect and lead to a total loss of control over eating.

Here's an example of how this works. Let's say you decide to stop eating your usual breakfast as a way to lose weight quickly. Cutting out a meal a day does save a lot of calories. Numerous studies, though, have shown that skipping meals is neither healthy nor an effective weight-loss method. Breakfast supplies important nutrients, so skipping this meal robs the body of the nutrients it needs for the morning and the rest of the day. Not surprisingly, the body often rebels with extreme hunger later in the morning. By lunchtime, excess hunger leads to overeating. Or, worse yet, the morning's hunger gets satisfied with a midmorning pastry. The body is still trying to make up the lost calories at dinnertime, and overeating continues.

# *Personal Triumph*

## Jeanne Lemoine

LOUISIANA

Jeanne Lemoine, a school system clerk, was very heavy even as an infant. As a child, she developed serious asthma and was treated with steroids and other medications that contributed to ongoing weight gain. Jeanne joined Weight Watchers as an adult and lost 99 pounds to reach her goal weight.

"I prefer to weigh in every week. My natural tendency is to stay within tight boundaries, to look for perfection. But now if I make a mistake, I just stand up, dust myself off, and keep going. I find that I can eat whatever I want as long as I keep track of what I'm eating. That's the method that works for me. In restaurants, I'm not afraid to ask how things are cooked and ask them to make adjustments for me.

"There were times when I didn't lose weight. My strategy was to write down what I ate and then review it to see what I could do differently. When I started with physical activity, I began with a walk around the park. I couldn't make it halfway around, I had to sit on every bench to regain my breath, and I had to use an inhaler for my asthma. Now I walk 4 miles easily, I exercise regularly, and I swim. Whenever I try a new activity, I start slowly and gradually build up. I am a firm believer in pacing weight loss. Taking it off quickly doesn't work."

*"I am a firm believer in pacing weight loss. Taking it off quickly doesn't work."*

Extreme weight-loss methods are difficult if not impossible to sustain for a long enough period of time to lose a significant amount of weight because they do not mesh with the realities of most people's lives. When people go back to their regular routines, all of their underlying issues related to weight management come back and create the same combustible mix that caused weight gain in the first place. It is far better to adopt a strategy of multiple steps that can be incorporated into the routines of daily life rather than choose a course of dramatic sacrifice and restriction that is likely to lead to rebound.

The opposite is also true. Flexible control—adjusting eating from meal to meal—is associated with a greater chance of losing weight successfully. Learning to regulate eating in a flexible way in sync with daily life probably helps explain why the establishment of a normal diet is a success factor for long-term weight loss.

Participants in the Weight Watchers LTM Database and the National Weight Control Registry (NWCR) report that they pay ongoing attention to what they eat and are conscious of their eating patterns without turning their lives upside down. They have found the balance among sensible eating, structure, and flexibility, with just enough structure to create consistency and enough flexibility to allow for choices from a wide variety of foods and in all kinds of social situations. Making conscious choices and being aware of what you are eating is the foundation for making wise food choices long term.

## Small Steps Toward Change

A central theme in this book is that of positive lifestyle and livability—that weight management has to fit your lifestyle and be something you can live with over time. The reason for focusing on this theme is simple. Study after study has shown that if people are asked to make extreme changes for fast weight loss, they simply cannot sustain the disruption. It is far better to take small steps toward new habits, fine-tuning daily practices to slowly incorporate them into your lifestyle. Using this strategy, weight management efforts can slowly and subtly become a part of your day-to-day life without disruption. This is the only proven way of sustaining weight loss for the long term.

Don't change everything at once. Our recommended approach is to start with a diet that provides all the essential nutrients and produces the desirable rate of weight loss. Incorporate and master diet changes first. Then, as your weight loss progresses and new eating habits become second nature to you, add physical activity and exercise to help minimize muscle loss and aid in maintaining the existing weight loss. The ultimate goal is steady, incremental weight loss of no more than 1 to 2 pounds per week maintained over time after the initial water weight loss of the first few weeks. This rate can be achieved without resorting to an extreme diet.

Progressive, stepwise changes in your food choices, eating patterns, and exercise habits produce this preferred rate of weight loss. Because they become part of your daily routine, you're better able to keep doing them for the long term.

## Keeping the Weight Off

The key to keeping the weight off is integrating into your daily life the skills and habits that you used while losing weight. This approach eases the transition between weight loss and keeping the weight off. If you have learned how to make consistently wise food choices, the foods and the social occasions that are part of daily life are not as big a challenge. You will have learned the skill of flexible control and will know what you need to do to enjoy the food that is part of special occasions while keeping the weight off.

Nipping small gains in the bud makes a difference. Research from the National Weight Control Registry (NWCR) found that the more weight that is regained, the harder it is to get back to your goal. In a large study that looked at diet, weight loss, and heart disease, the researchers found that a weight gain of 5 pounds is predictive of long-term weight gain.

Making lifestyle changes and successfully losing weight do not guarantee that the process of coping with life's challenges will not lead you to regain some of the weight back. Life is full of stressful times, like planning a wedding, raising children, having extra demands placed on you at work, or losing a job or a loved one. Just as the Institute of Medicine (IOM) outlined predictors of successful weight maintenance, its report also listed factors leading to weight regain, including negative life events and family dysfunction.

The key is to realize this and to take action as soon as you are able. The sooner you are able to get back on track, the greater success you will have.

## The Physical Factor

Successful, sustainable weight loss is not only about how many calories you eat or establishing a style of flexible control. In a review of the research that compared moderate- and low-calorie diets, it was concluded that regardless of the calorie level of the diet used to lose weight, regular exercise, participation in a formal weight-loss maintenance program, or both are likely to achieve the best long-term results.

Let's look at physical activity as an integral part of long-term weight loss. It is important to avoid the extreme of trying to do too much exercise too quickly if you have not been active on a regular basis. Going from no activity to a plan to jog daily is too ambitious!

For the vast majority of people who either have been inactive or have gained weight, the best strategy is to start with a program of walking, maybe just ten or so minutes per day (see chapter 4 for more detailed guidelines). An intermediate goal might be to follow the recommendations of the Centers for Disease Control to try to accumulate thirty minutes of moderate-intensity physical activity on most if not all days. Once you've achieved this goal, you'll know that you're getting the health benefits that regular activity can provide.

The key words are *accumulate* and *moderate*. The activity you choose should not be so intense that it leaves you breathless or unable to

# *Personal Triumph*

## Lori Anthony

NEW ENGLAND

Lori Anthony, a market data specialist, always struggled with her weight. She is now 3 pounds away from her goal weight, having lost 113 pounds.

"My weight went way up when I was pregnant with my second child, and I didn't take any of it off. I tried so many different diets but just gained the weight back. When I joined Weight Watchers, I was so heavy that most activity was difficult for me. My first goal was to walk around the block. Once I accomplished that, I set new goals to walk farther. Eventually, I got into a routine of walking up to 4 miles three or four times weekly. Believe it or not, that started feeling too much like recreation.

*"Now I truly enjoy life. I can enjoy sun-filled days outside rather than hiding in the house."*

"Last summer, I joined a gym and started working with a personal trainer. I also take exercise classes. The biggest benefit from becoming more active is that I now enjoy going out and taking a walk. I never expected myself to want to do that; I never wanted to do any type of activity. Now I truly enjoy life. I can enjoy sun-filled days outside rather than hiding in the house."

speak while you exercise. The goal is to establish a consistent, pleasurable level of physical activity in your daily life. As physical activity becomes part of your routine, shoot for the exercise recommendation for people who are sustaining weight loss: sixty to ninety minutes of moderate-intensity activity per day.

## The Mind Matters

Your mind is a powerful ally in your quest for long-term weight loss. With the proper knowledge and attitude, the mind can work with the body to create positive new behaviors. Here's how:

1. Set a realistic goal or a combination of short-, intermediate-, and long-term goals. For example, a short-term goal might be to lose 10% of your current weight. A longer-term goal might be to sustain the weight loss for at least six months.
2. Break your goals into smaller action steps.
3. Do a confidence check: Do you believe that you can achieve your goals? If yes, keep going. If no, set new goals that are more attainable.
4. Have frequent pep rallies to boost your spirit. Be your own cheerleader and enlist others to cheer with you. Tell yourself often and loudly that you can do it. Think about how good you felt when you achieved your goals in the past. Believe in yourself and see the results.
5. Visualize yourself doing positive new behaviors, like asking for food the way you want it at a restaurant. Continue to visualize what you can accomplish and the benefits that will come with sustained weight loss.
6. Come up with new strategies if your initial ones are not working or are not working as well as they were.
7. Recognize and give yourself credit for the gains you've already made. Compliment yourself. Think positively about your good

qualities and successes, rather than drawing on or dwelling on negative thoughts.

8. Reward yourself with nonfood rewards, like an evening at the movies or an afternoon with a friend, for reaching a goal or successfully changing a behavior.

## The Bottom Line

The method used to lose weight makes a big difference in achieving weight loss that lasts. Extreme methods may produce fast weight loss, but they don't provide weight loss that lasts. Many participants in the Weight Watchers LTM Database and NWCR say that they lost and gained weight many times using extreme methods. It was only when they ultimately recognized the truth—long-term, sustainable weight loss requires a comprehensive weight-loss method that is realistic, livable, and sustainable—that they achieved their desired outcome of successful weight loss.

# Personal Triumph

## Katherine Deliso

MASSACHUSETTS

Katherine Deliso, a librarian, says, "My weight gain began when I was about 25. I used to be able to eat whatever I wanted. Then the pounds started piling on. I started graduate school and I really started gaining weight because I was eating during studying. Then a personal trauma hit and I started eating even more. When I hit size 18 and realized that I could get to 200 pounds, I knew I had to do something and joined Weight Watchers. I set a goal weight of 130 pounds but realized that it was too low for me.

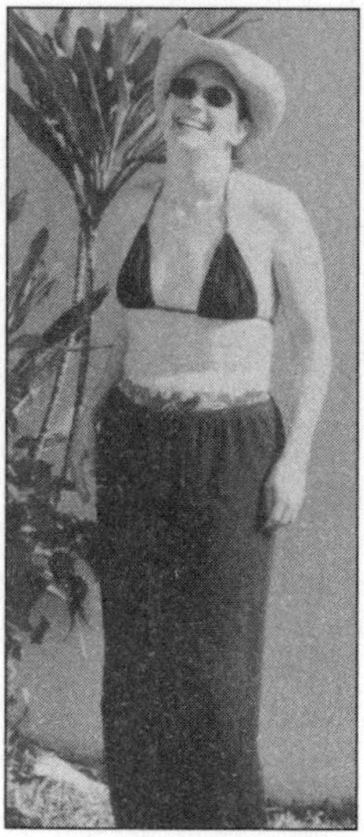

"My weight fluctuates a lot between the beginning of the month and the end of the month, so I had to raise my goal weight a bit. Setting a more realistic goal helped prevent me from getting frustrated. It also encourages me because my weight is almost always below my goal now. I also remind myself that I dropped five dress sizes. That is a lot. Thinking about that boosts my self-esteem and helps keep me on track."

*"Setting a more realistic goal helped prevent me from getting frustrated."*

Katherine lost 50 pounds.

## Weight Loss That Lasts

# Action Steps

Evaluating any weight-loss method you are considering to see if it is comprehensive, healthy, livable, and sustainable is time well spent.

- Remind yourself that weight loss that lasts is better than quickly losing and regaining the same 20 pounds over and over again. Avoiding extreme methods will help you get off the roller coaster.
- Pace your weight loss to a rate of 1 to 2 pounds per week. Enjoy the bigger weight loss that you're likely to see in the first couple of weeks, but know that it is water weight and that you're doing the right thing by pacing your weight loss for the longer term.
- Once you've achieved your weight goal, monitor your weight on a regular basis. Take prompt action if your weight gain reaches the 5-pound mark.

# Chapter 9

## Is there one right approach to weight loss?

To judge by the aisles at the local bookstore or the infomercials on television, there is a new and ultimate solution for weight loss every week. At least one weight-loss book usually is on the bestseller list along with sequels and companion books to former bestsellers. Many claim they have discovered the breakthrough to the mystery of weight loss and that their new discovery will work for everyone.

This chapter explores the myth that there is one simple solution to weight loss that will work for everyone. You will learn that there are ways to sort out the facts from the fiction.

# Myth 9 There is only one right approach to losing weight

*Believers Beware!*

There is a right weight-loss approach that everyone can follow and be guaranteed to lose weight. The latest hot diet book has discovered a revolutionary approach to lose weight. The discovery is based on new science that proves when it comes to losing weight, calories do not matter. The reason you have not been successful in losing weight in the past is that you have bought into the calorie myth and it is false. The latest hot diet book dispels this notion and puts you on the path to shedding those unwanted pounds. What's more, your weight loss happens with little or no effort on your part because it is the new scientific breakthrough that makes the weight come off.

The idea of a scientific breakthrough is very promising. After all, think of all of the new drugs and medical treatments that we hear about almost daily that have changed the lives of all the people who have tried them. If it can happen in those areas, it can happen in weight loss as well. And even if this week's version does not turn out to be the ultimate answer, it's worth trying. It might just work. You will never know unless you try.

Advertisements on television and in magazines say that new diets and products work. Many guarantee your success and will give you your money back if you don't lose all the weight you want. They wouldn't be able to make these promises if they didn't have scientific proof and the success to back them up.

## Kernels of Truth

It is not surprising that many people are looking for a new and different approach to losing weight. People tend to look for a new approach whenever the one that they were using before did not work. Even if the approach got them to lose weight, it did not last. Several surveys have shown that just about every person who has tried to lose weight—and that is a lot of people—has tried a variety of different approaches.

In one survey of adults, a general diet and exercise approach was the most frequently used method for both men and women, followed by vitamins, meal replacements, over-the-counter products, participation in a weight-loss program, and diet supplements. In another survey focusing on younger people, skipping meals was a method used by almost half of all women (interestingly, men did not seem to employ this method). With so many approaches to try, the idea of a new and different one not only makes sense, it is appealing.

The science of weight management as we know it is only about fifty years old, a baby in the world of science. In the early 1960s, *therapeutic starvation* was the treatment of choice. This particularly diabolical trend was followed by low-calorie diets that restricted particular foods, then moved on to protein-sparing modified fasts that took the idea of food completely out of the weight-loss equation. If you are more than a few decades old, you probably remember these approaches and can attest to the fact that they rarely resulted in sustained weight loss.

Fortunately, the science of weight management has advanced over the years. Dr. Albert Stunkard, the researcher who said back in the 1950s that 95% of diets fail, frequently talks about the advances that have been made in weight management treatments since he put forth his discouraging statistic over fifty years ago. In an article he published in the 1990s on the topic in the prestigious *American Journal of Medicine*, Dr. Stunkard attributes the advances to the recognition that a variety of factors must be included in a comprehensive weight-loss program. He also credits improved weight-loss success rates to the realization that weight management cannot be viewed as a one-time, weight-loss event that disappears with the achievement of a weight goal. It is not the same as completing a course of antibiotics to get rid of a bacterial infection. Rather, sustained weight loss involves making ongoing lifestyle changes.

## The Whole Truth

The central theme of this book is that weight loss that lasts requires a comprehensive method including making wise food choices, getting more active, making positive lifestyle changes, and creating a supportive atmosphere.

This chapter focuses on making wise food choices. Most weight-loss methods address only this component of weight loss, and it is an important one. But you might be wondering how to choose from the hundreds of food plans out there.

**Three Steps to Finding the Right Approach for You**

Start with the hundreds of diets that are available, then ask yourself:

1. Does it create a calorie deficit?
2. Is it healthy?
3. Does it fit my life?

If you answer yes to all these questions, it's the one for you!

### Weight Loss Means Cutting Calories, and There Are Many Ways to Do It

The fundamental scientific truth of weight loss is that it can occur if a caloric deficit is created. This is the first question when considering any weight-loss method. To lose a pound of fat "costs" about 3,500 calories and those calories have to be "paid" by eating fewer calories than the body needs to stay the way it is, by burning more calories than the

# *Personal Triumph*

## Charlotte Miller

MINNESOTA

Charlotte Miller, a gift shop employee, lost over 40 pounds to reach her goal weight. She had lost weight successfully on Weight Watchers in the 1980s but gained all the weight back when she stopped following the program. In the interim, Charlotte tried other programs but eventually rejoined Weight Watchers. Now that she has reached her goal weight, Charlotte continues to weigh in at a Weight Watchers meeting at least once per month.

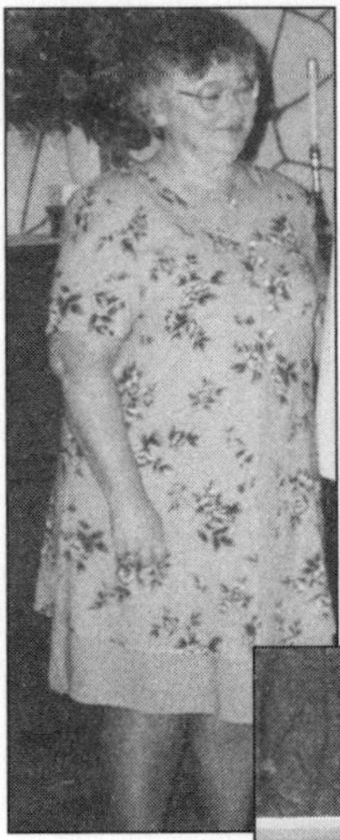

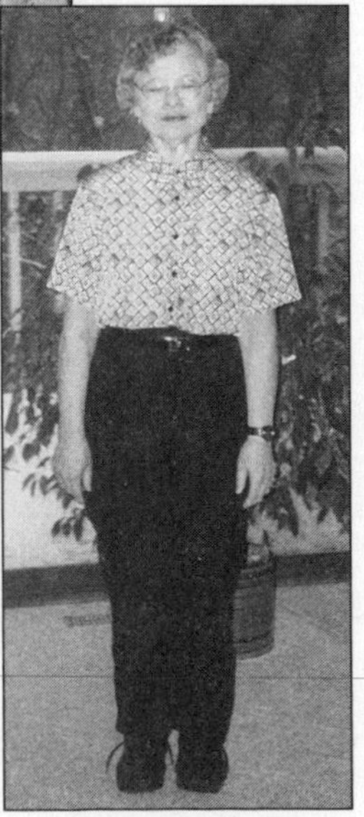

"Those monthly weigh-ins help me monitor myself and hold me accountable for any changes in my weight from month to month."

*"Those monthly weigh-ins help me monitor myself and hold me accountable for any changes in my weight from month to month."*

body needs to stay the way it is, or a combination of the two. But the number of approaches that a person can take to create the caloric deficit is infinite.

Then, the question is whether the food plan is healthy. Is it nutritionally complete? Does it encourage healthy eating habits? It is possible to eat just enough bacon or chocolate-chip cookies during the whole day to create the calorie deficit you need to lose weight. But your goal is to get your essential nutrition from healthy meals from *all* the food groups.

Because you are a unique individual with your own personality, lifestyle, preferences, and eating style, the path you follow to achieve sustained weight loss must be your own. The notion of a single approach that works for everyone could hold true only if we were all the same. The laws of thermodynamics for weight loss are universal (1 pound of fat = 3,500 calories), but the laws of human nature (no two human beings are identical) hold true as well.

To lose weight and keep it off, it is critical to find the approach that is right for you. Does the eating plan fit your preferences and your lifestyle? Does is it encourage healthy eating habits you can keep up? Counting and writing down calories is an effective approach to self-monitoring food intake for many people, but that does not mean that it is right for everyone. For some people, finding another mechanism that will ensure they eat fewer calories than they burn is preferable. The guideline is to monitor food intake—the approach of how this is done varies.

The focus of credible weight management research today is to define and refine the factors that are critical in a comprehensive weight-loss program, then provide a set of guidelines that reflect the findings. For example, the preponderance of evidence shows that about sixty to ninety minutes of moderate physical activity per day is associated with sustained weight loss. Science does not say that the exercise has to be walking or swimming or that it has to be done in a single session or spread throughout the day. Your approach is *how* you create the caloric deficit needed to lose weight.

The remainder of this chapter explores some of the most important things for you to consider in sorting through the myriad available weight-loss approaches.

### Wonder Diets Are One-Hit Wonders

It is safe to predict that at least one new wonder diet or product will be promoted this year. It is also safe to predict that next year and the year after that will bring new wonder diets and products. The trend has been well established. A recent online search of books under the title or topic of weight loss revealed 2,214 matches! As the problem of excess weight has increased in the United States and around the developed world, the proliferation of diet books has followed suit.

Every year, new diet books promise a revolutionary approach to weight-loss success. Call these one-diet wonders, much like the one-hit wonder bands in popular music that release one hit song and rarely are heard from again. Like the one-hit wonder bands, these diets come onto the weight-loss scene with a splash. Devotees gush over the new diets. But like hit songs and bands, new diets and their creators vanish quickly once the reality of short-term weight loss overtakes the promise of thinness forever.

Most bestsellers do not last, whether they are songs or books. According to a conference report from the National Arts Journalism Program at Columbia University, most diet bestsellers do not stand the test of time. They are on the shelf today and out of print only a few years later. Trendy ideas in weight loss change very quickly and do not make for true longevity.

## Testimonials Are One Person's Story

Almost any approach to weight loss will work for at least one person. Every approach can offer testimonials about how it led to weight loss. While motivating and fun, testimonials need to be read with caution. If the testimonial is one example of the real-world success of many people who have followed the diet, then it can be a valuable resource. But

# Personal Triumph

## Jeanne Lemoine

LOUISIANA

Jeanne Lemoine, whom we introduced in chapter 8, admits that she was so heavy that she could not cross one leg over the other while sitting in a chair. She tried to lose weight several times before she joined Weight Watchers.

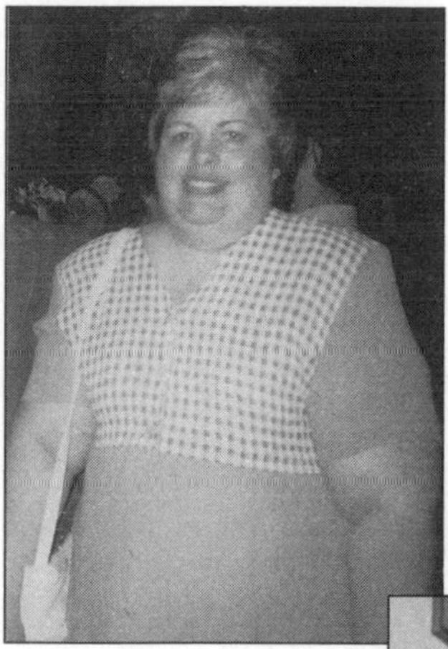

"Weight Watchers doesn't feel like a diet. That is the difference between the program and fad diets. On Weight Watchers, I can eat the way I want to eat. Weight Watchers offers tremendous variety.

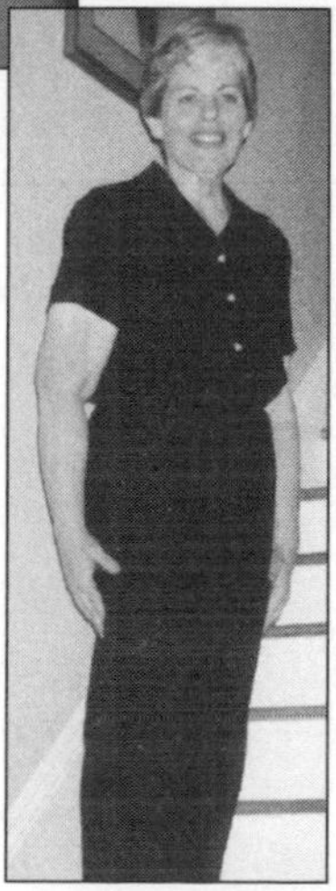

"When I'm out, I bring along my program materials so that I can figure out how any food can fit into my diet. I write everything down in a notebook so that I can monitor my eating and find any problem spots. This was especially important when I was trying to lose weight and hitting plateaus. My journal showed me where I had strayed."

*"On Weight Watchers, I can eat the way I want to eat. Weight Watchers offers tremendous variety."*

testimonials are just one piece of the evaluation process. They are usually most helpful for learning about the practical aspects of a weight-loss method—which foods are encouraged or discouraged, tips for following the recommended approach to eating, and how making the recommended changes affected the person's life. They are only useful if they go beyond headlines like "I lost 50 pounds in one month."

## Sort the Truth from the Fiction

Most new diet approaches are simply nonsense, although some are legitimate. Unfortunately, at times it can even be difficult for health professionals to tell the difference because scientific explanations that sound so believable. What are some of the tricks for spotting short-term fixes? Typically, they are promoted with grand words like "revolutionary" or "miracle." Beneath their title, they often include a tag line with an appealing promise, such as "based on a scientific breakthrough" or "the only program you will ever need." The front or back cover of the book will include other appealing promises: "lose weight forever," "never be hungry," "drop pounds quickly and painlessly." When it comes to weight-loss promises, if it sounds too good to be true, it often is too good to be true.

Public health organizations have become more active in helping people make informed choices about weight loss. Overweight is a big problem, and the potential for harm or good has greatly increased. Organizations like the American Heart Association (AHA) and the American Dietetic Association, as well as government agencies like the National Institutes of Health and the Federal Trade Commission, provide information and resources to help people sort through the many options available to them.

AHA has declared war on fad diets. As part of its comprehensive education campaign, AHA provides information to help identify ineffective or questionable weight-loss diets and claims. AHA discourages following programs that do not advise people with diabetes, high blood pressure, or other long-term health problems to seek advice from their physician or other health care provider. It also disapproves of programs and diets that do not call for increased physical activity and specifically cautions against certain types of fad diets.

**The American Heart Association Does Not Endorse:**

Specific combinations of foods or food combining
Diets that eliminate dairy
Liquid-only diets
Programs that require the purchase of packaged meals
High-protein diets
Juice fasting
"Cleansing" diets
Bizarre quantities of only one food (hot dogs, cabbage soup)
Magic or miracle foods that burn fat
Rigid menus with limited foods
Rapid weight loss of more than 2 pounds a week

*Source:* Adapted from www.americanheart.org.

## Find Credible Resources

Armed with strategies for sorting out truth from fiction, it is time to turn to credible resources for information on weight control. According to the government's National Institutes of Health Weight-Control Information Network (WIN), "Experts agree that the best way to reach a healthy weight is to follow a sensible eating plan and engage in regular physical activity. Weight-loss programs should encourage healthy behaviors that help you lose weight and that you can maintain over time." Because activity is covered more fully in chapter 4, this chapter will focus on what to look for in the food plan of a comprehensive weight-loss program.

A credible source for weight-loss information is the Partnership for Healthy Weight Management. Coordinated by the government's Federal Trade Commission, the mission of this partnership is to promote sound guidance on strategies for achieving and maintaining a healthy weight. A core principle of the partnership is that no single weight-loss approach will work for everyone. The partnership offers general guidance that is in agreement with the principles in this book: nutritional balance, nutrient intake consistent with recommendations for health promotion and disease prevention, and a rate of weight loss that promotes loss of body fat rather than lean muscle. Its brochure available at www.ftc.gov/bcp/conline/pubs/health/wgtloss.pdf includes a personal checklist for helping select a weight-loss method in line with the partnership's mission.

**Questions to Ask When Choosing a Food Plan**

Does it encourage sensible, balanced eating?

Does it include foods from all food groups?

Does it meet all my nutrient needs?

Does it provide information on healthy eating?

## Consider Other Factors

In addition to the general factors promoted by the Partnership for Healthy Weight Management, these other factors should be considered when evaluating a weight-loss food plan

*Is the plan clear and up front about the role of calories in weight loss?* Experts agree that the overwhelming driver of weight loss is the creation of a caloric deficit—fewer calories in than out. No good scientific proof of any kind supports changes in metabolism or other magic approaches to melt away body fat.

*Does the plan support an eating pattern that fits your individual lifestyle*

*and preferences?* Eating plans are easier to follow when they fit the dieter's lifestyle and include foods that the dieter enjoys eating. Recently, the AHA revised its dietary guidelines to emphasize the importance of flexibility in food selection.

The number of daily meals and snacks should be based on personal preference. There is no right or wrong approach when it comes to a plan with three meals and a snack versus six or so mini-meals per day. People who have a low level of dietary restraint and respond to food cues by being tempted to eat or overeat may prefer fewer meals and snacks in order to minimize exposure to food. Using an extreme method like skipping meals is not recommended, and eating in an overly strict way to comply with a specific method is not, either.

*Does the plan give eating satisfaction?* Eating provides pleasure, so you want to enjoy the food that you are eating both while you are losing weight and while you are keeping the weight off. Eating satisfaction is a complex issue, and there is no one meal plan or eating style that is satisfying for everyone.

*Have you ever heard . . .*

**"You have to eat breakfast if you want to lose weight."**

Eating breakfast or skipping breakfast will not directly lead to weight loss or gain. However, eating breakfast is likely to affect overall caloric intake for the day. And when it comes to the research, the findings about breakfast are pretty clear: people who eat a light breakfast (for example, cereal and fruit) weigh less than people who skip breakfast or have a heavy breakfast (for example, eggs and bacon). Eating breakfast is also an approach shared by the vast majority of National Weight Control Registry (NWCR) volunteers, with only 4% saying that they never eat breakfast.

## Factors Affecting Eating Satisfaction

Eating satisfaction is linked to a variety of factors. What works for one person when it comes to eating satisfaction may not work for another. Finding what works is key because being satisfied affects the ability to lose weight and keep it off. While there is no single formula for eating satisfaction, there are threads that can guide you toward finding the pattern that works best.

Body processes involved in the regulation of appetite are very complex and involve a number of hormones and biological systems. Other factors that affect eating satisfaction include taste, palatability, and energy density. Likewise, the composition of food affects eating satisfaction. In general, high-protein foods are more satisfying than foods with carbohydrates, and carbohydrate foods are more satisfying than high-fat foods. Alcohol stimulates eating.

The term *carbohydrate* encompasses thousands of foods from sugar to wheat germ. The effect of carbohydrates on eating satisfaction varies. Research suggests that whole grains provide greater eating satisfaction than refined grains. Dietary fiber, a component of carbohydrate foods, has been shown to reduce hunger and increase satiety. Increasing fiber intake as a weight-loss strategy appears to be related to the amount of excess weight—the more weight to lose, the more effective the strategy.

Energy density plays a role too. Some recent research has shown that from a very young age, people are trained to eat a volume of food, not a certain amount of calories. For example, most people will fill the same bowl every time they eat soup; they will not fill the bowl less full if it is a high-calorie bisque or have a second bowl if it is a low-calorie broth. An effective approach to reduce caloric intake is to choose foods with a low energy density because the amount of food that can be eaten for a set number of calories is greater for a low-energy-density food than it is for a high-energy-density food. In other words, you get more food for the calories, and more food is associated with higher eating satisfaction.

For example, a cup of boiled corn is 130 calories. A cup of air-popped popcorn is 30 calories. Both are kernels of corn, but with popcorn the kernel has been pumped up with air and that makes popcorn a low-energy-density food that is low in calories.

Foods with a low energy density increase eating satisfaction with fewer calories because these foods usually are higher in water or air, lower in fat, and/or higher in fiber. Fruits and vegetables, for example, are rich in water and fiber. As such, they are low-energy-density foods that are useful for weight management. A review of studies looking at weight loss over at least six months concluded that a dietary pattern lower in fat and higher in fiber provided the best results.

For the same calories, a portion of a low-energy-density food is larger than a higher-density food portion. High-energy-density foods, many of which are concentrated sources of refined carbohydrates, sugars, and/or fat and taste good, are more likely to be overeaten. They are harder to stop eating in a single setting and over time.

Several studies have looked at whether altering the amount of food provided or altering the calories in the amount of food makes people eat differently. The findings are consistent. The daily amount of food eaten influences appetite; the number of calories eaten does not affect appetite.

## Self-Monitor to Stay on Track

Finding an eating pattern and foods that provide eating satisfaction are critical to lasting weight loss because eating in a way that works for you enables you to stay the course. But there is one more component that is essential: self-monitoring. Without a system in place that helps you monitor what you are doing and eating, it is easy to stray off the path of weight loss and return to old habits without even realizing it. Several studies have found that self-monitoring makes a significant difference when it comes to successful weight loss. One study showed that 25% of weight-loss success is attributable to consistent self-monitoring. The people who are the most consistent in self-monitoring have the greatest success.

There is no right or wrong way to self-monitor. Self-monitoring takes different forms and measures different things. It works when you find a method that you are comfortable with and are willing to do over time.

Most people benefit from monitoring two separate but related things when it comes to weight loss: food intake and body weight. Tracking food intake can be as simple as counting and writing down some measurement of food eaten, for example, calories or ***POINTS*** values of foods. Tracking may be expanded to include recording the food item and the portion that is eaten in addition to its calorie or ***POINTS*** information. To add even more detail, the tracking can include information about what time of day a food is eaten and/or feelings experienced while eating. Information can be written down on a piece of note paper, on an index card, or in a journal, whichever is most convenient.

When used consistently, tracking food intake in writing produces superior weight-loss results. However, not all dieters are consistent in their short-term tracking and over time.

Assessing internal cues for and feelings of hunger and satiety is an alternative method of monitoring eating habits and patterns and eating satisfaction. In practical terms, this means eating the amount of food needed for eating satisfaction, then stopping. Internal cues are closely linked with the person's level of dietary restraint and disinhibition (see chapter 3 for a more detailed discussion). One theory says that overweight people do not recognize their body's cues for hunger or satiety because they never learned how to do this. Learning to recognize and self-monitor these cues may be a helpful technique in weight management.

Monitoring food intake helps keep track of the weight-loss *process;* monitoring weight loss keeps track of weight-loss *progress*. Weight loss can be monitored in several different ways: body weight, body measurements, or the clothing test.

Body weight is the easiest measure of progress. An added benefit of using weighing as a self-monitoring strategy is that it allows pacing of weight loss to equal a 1- to 2-pound loss weekly. Body weight measurement is more effective as a weekly weigh-in than as a daily weigh-in. Because body weight fluctuates a great deal from day to day for many reasons, including menstrual status and recent sodium and carbohydrate intake, it is easy to put too much stock into a change, be it up or down, with a daily weigh-in. A weekly weigh-in is a better indicator of true weight-loss progress and trends.

Body measurements are an alternative to weighing, especially for people who feel stressed from watching the scale numbers go down and up. Keep measurements simple by sticking to key body parts like the bust, waist, and hips. Because measurements change more slowly than weight does, body measurements should be taken only once a month or so.

The clothing test is the simplest method of self-monitoring. One way to do the clothing test is to monitor the fit of a favorite pair of pants or a favorite nonstretch shirt. Try the clothing on immediately after washing before it stretches out with wear. The belt-notch test is particularly useful for men.

Monitoring your weight-loss progress can be a solo event or it can be done with someone's help. Some people find that being accountable to others is useful. Accountability can include weighing in weekly with a spouse or partner, participating in a structured weight-loss program that includes monitoring activities as part of its program (such as being weighed each week by trained staff), or having a monthly appointment with a physician or health professional to assess your progress. Regardless of the monitoring method chosen, the goal of keeping track is to learn how it's working.

At the end of the day, paced weight loss is the yardstick for success and goal attainment. And, as shown in the Institute of Medicine (IOM) report and the National Weight Control Registry (NWCR) database, regular monitoring is key to keeping the weight off. The IOM report lists self-monitoring as a positive predictor of weight loss as well as maintenance of weight loss. Participants in the NWCR database say that they frequently monitor their food intake and their body weight.

# *Personal Triumph*

**Shelli Beers**
MARYLAND

Shelli Beers, whom we met in chapter 6, explains, "One morning, I couldn't fit into any of my pairs of pants, and I just sat on the floor and cried. That day I went to work and talked to a couple of my coworkers who had lost a lot of weight on Weight Watchers. I decided it was better to spend money on Weight Watchers than on even bigger pairs of pants, so I joined.

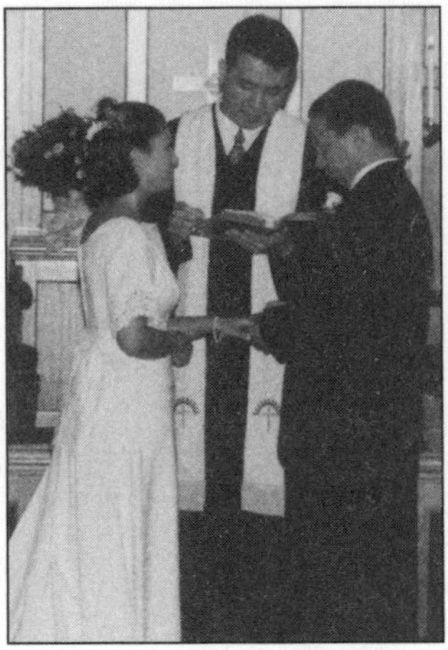

"When I first started Weight Watchers, I was scared to death of that scale. In the past, it never had good news for me. But weighing every week at Weight Watchers meetings helped me overcome my fear of the scale and helped me learn that the scale is my accountability and my friend. Weighing in tells me how I am doing week to week."

*"Weighing in tells me how I am doing week to week."*

The first time Shelli got married, she wanted to wear her mother's wedding gown but could not fit into it. She lost 56 pounds to her goal weight and wore the dress for her second wedding.

## The Bottom Line

When it comes to weight loss, one diet or approach does not fit all. While there are many ways you can create a calorie deficit, you should also choose a food plan based on whether it is healthy and a good fit with your preferences and lifestyle. We all are different, with different personal habits and preferences. That is why what works for one person may not work or be the right approach for someone else. The science of weight management continues to evolve as researchers learn which program elements help people sustain their weight loss.

Beware of being lured into trying the latest and greatest diets. They usually sound terrific and make big promises. Keep in mind that testimonials, as convincing as they sound, do not apply to everyone and may not tell the full story. Enjoy success stories as a way to get inspired and find out what following the weight-loss program might be like for you. Remember that many diet programs have not been proven with large numbers of people and have not passed the test of time for lasting weight loss.

It is important to look carefully at weight-loss programs for proof that they are healthy and that they work. Compare their features to those discussed by the American Heart Association and use the Partnership for Healthy Weight Management for guidance on selecting an appropriate program. Important features for effective weight loss include adaptability to individual lifestyle and preferences and a diet that is satisfying to eat.

Self-monitoring is essential. Monitoring eating habits and weight loss helps track the process and progress of weight loss. There is no right or wrong way to self-monitor, as long as it is sustainable and useful. Self-monitoring enables you to make adjustments in eating habits for a desirable pace of weight loss.

# Weight Loss That Lasts
# Action Steps

There are so many weight-loss approaches, yet most of us have very little time to do a complete evaluation. The good news is that a cursory evaluation can weed out the ones that have no value. From there, you can try out one or several.

- Review credible Web sites and information sources on sensible weight-loss programs to remind yourself of features to look for.
- Adjust your daily meal schedule to fit your lifestyle and ability to handle your food cues.
- Include foods that provide you with eating satisfaction that fit into your recommended eating plan.
- Find self-monitoring tools that work for you: a journal, a tape measure, a high-quality bathroom scale, or a piece of clothing to measure yourself.
- If you are weighing yourself, try to be consistent with the day of week, time of day, and clothing (or not) that you are wearing.
- Use the results of your weight-loss monitoring (body weight and/or body size) to help you make changes to your program. If your weight loss exceeds 2 pounds per week, eat a bit more and keep monitoring. If your weight loss is less than 1 pound per week, adjust your food intake slightly downward, evaluate your food choices and focus more on lower-energy-density foods, and/or increase your physical activity.

# Chapter 10

# Is my weight problem just about me?

Many people think about their weight in an isolated way, focusing only on how their weight affects their well-being and what they themselves can do to manage their weight. They ignore or don't pay attention to how the way they deal with their weight affects the people around them and how those people are helping or hurting what they are trying to accomplish.

This chapter explores the realities of the "it's only about me" weight management myth. You will discover how you can help people you care about and how you can enlist people around you to help you.

# Myth 10 Your weight is your problem and you need to solve it on your own

*Believers Beware!*

Weight is a personal matter, and the decisions a person makes about it are personal choices. The people with whom you live, including partners and children, are unaffected by your weight and weight issues. This holds true whether you are overweight and not doing anything about it or if you are losing weight. Likewise, if the choice is made to lose weight, it is a path that is best walked alone. The person who wants to lose weight has to make the commitment to do so and that commitment need not involve anyone else.

Losing weight is somewhat selfish since the person who loses the weight is the one who reaps all the benefits. Spouses, children, and friends are not really affected when you decide to make a change like losing weight. What they do won't help or hurt your weight loss.

## Kernels of Truth

Your weight is a part of who you are and as such it has a major impact on your quality of life. Each day, you interact with a lot of people—everyone from your partner to your family, friends, coworkers, acquaintances, even strangers. These are the relationships by which our lives as social beings are defined. And because your weight is a part of you, it also has an impact on your relationships with others. The effects can be positive, negative, or neutral.

Weight is a very personal matter. Regardless of how much they weigh, most people are reluctant to talk about this with anyone else, including those with whom they are intimate. Nobody likes to get on the scale at the doctor's office. Likewise, the decision to lose weight is a personal choice. No one can make the decision for you. It is only natural to feel that you are on your own when it comes to making decisions about weight.

The process of losing weight requires a personal commitment to accept responsibility for making the necessary lifestyle choices. Once weight is lost, continued commitment is needed to sustain the weight loss. These commitments are highly personal and cannot be made by anyone else. When it comes to losing weight and keeping it off, many people prefer to do it on their own.

Although this may work, it also makes the weight-loss process more challenging than it needs to be. Let's take a look at how your weight can affect you and your relationships as you travel the path to sustained weight loss.

## The Whole Truth

### You and Your Weight

You are probably familiar with the phrase *quality of life*. While it is a descriptive phrase that many of us use in the course of everyday conversation, it is also a term that researchers use to assess how a person is functioning in the course of his or her daily life. Just as there

# *Personal Triumph*

## Dianne Raynor

GEORGIA

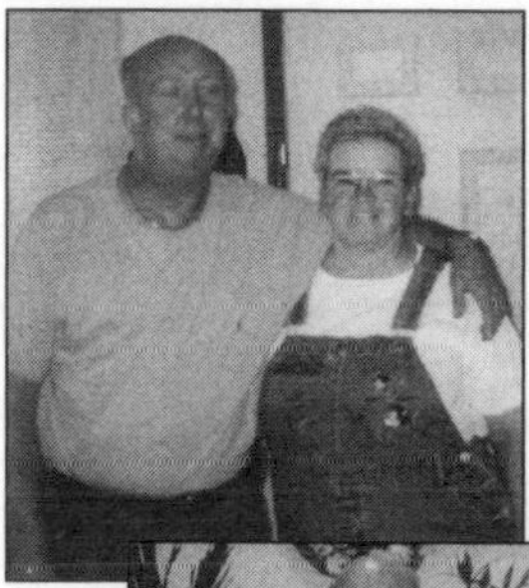

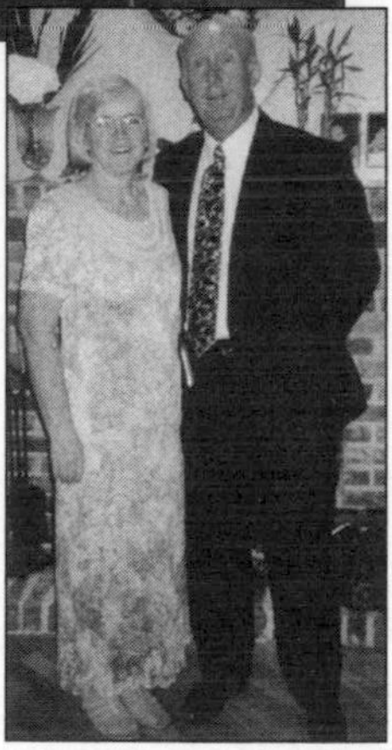

Dianne Raynor, a small business owner, battled her weight for many years. Eating was Dianne's cure-all for everything—nervousness, stress, boredom. Dianne joined Weight Watchers about twenty years ago and lost weight. Then she underwent several surgeries and gained weight again.

"I had high blood pressure and arthritis in my knee, and I couldn't walk more than fifteen minutes while shopping at the mall. I decided that I would die if I didn't lose weight, since many of my family members have serious health problems.

"My husband and I joined Weight Watchers together because he had gained weight since stopping smoking. Although I wanted to lose weight for me, not for anyone else, having the support of my husband made a big difference. I truly believe that Weight Watchers saved both of our lives. We support each other and we have a tremendous support system at our meetings.

"I feel so much better now! I no longer take medication for high blood pressure or arthritis. My doctor says that nobody would believe the change between my before and after health records."

*"My doctor says that nobody would believe the change between my before and after health records."*

One of Dianne's personal goals was to not have to buy clothing in the larger women's departments. She now shops in the petite department and even wears a smaller shoe size. Dianne lost 67 pounds to reach her goal weight.

are standard tests that are used to measure if your thyroid gland is functioning properly or if your cholesterol is normal, there are tests that measure *health-related quality of life*, or HRQL. There are many parts to the test, and several of the aspects that are measured can be influenced by weight. Examples of weight-related qualities include body pain, mental health, social functioning, physical limitations, fatigue, vigor, and feelings of vitality.

Many people are under the mistaken notion that every overweight person is depressed, sad, and unhappy with life. That simply is not true. A lot of studies have looked at these quality-of-life aspects in people who are overweight. In a study done in Italy, it was concluded that the greater the degree of overweight, the more negative the scores for physical functions like body pain, physical limitations, and fatigue. This makes sense because carrying extra weight around takes a toll on the body, and overweight and lack of physical fitness are closely connected. But the same Italian study also found that the impact of excess weight on mental status is minimal. Most experts agree that the psychological profile for the typical overweight person is not much different from that of her slimmer counterpart. As health care professionals working in the area of weight management, we talk with people every day who are happy, confident, and enjoying life. In fact, many come to us saying, "I am a together person who has every aspect of my life in order except my weight, and I am now making it my priority to get that under control too."

Where does this "all overweight people are unhappy" myth come from? Most likely, it is a misinterpretation of the medical literature. Many people with medically diagnosed eating disorders like bulimia nervosa are overweight. The issues at the root of eating disorders are psychological in nature; they are not about making wiser food choices and becoming more physically active. It is imperative that eating disorders be treated by mental health professionals.

In addition to eating disorders, there are people with severe morbid obesity whose weight has affected their life to such a great degree that they are psychologically unhealthy. Because this unique group of people has been extensively studied and reported on, they get portrayed as typical. Again, this is simply not the case.

If overweight people are not unhappy as a rule, is the reverse true? Are heavier people psychologically better off? That does not seem to be the case either. In a study done in Houston on residents over 50 years of age, eight aspects of mental health were assessed: happiness, perceived mental health, life satisfaction, positive affect, negative affect, optimism, feeling loved and cared for, and depression. None of these factors showed higher scores for subjects who were overweight. Either weight did not make a difference or the heaviest residents were a little worse off.

Just as researchers have looked at the impact of quality-of-life factors on being overweight, many studies have been done to evaluate if there are changes in the test scores when weight is lost. This is where the story changes. Just about every study shows that several aspects of life quality improve with weight loss. In a twelve-week study conducted by Dr. Rippe and his colleagues on people participating in the Weight Watchers program, several measures of quality of life—including physical function, vitality, and mental health—improved with weight loss. Participants were less fatigued and had greater feelings of vigor as a result of participating in the study.

While simply losing weight improves the quality of life, the method by which weight is lost also has an impact. A weight-loss program that includes making positive lifestyle changes and a supportive atmosphere in addition to focusing on food and exercise changes makes a difference in quality scores. In one study that included all of these components, participants lost an average of 20 pounds, improved their scores by 5% to 19%, and reported a significant improvement in how healthy they felt.

Weight loss improves the physical health aspects of life quality because the body does not have to work as hard when it is not required to carry excess weight around. Weight loss also has a positive impact on mood, which, in turn improves your mental health. *These improvements in physical and mental functioning have a positive impact on the relationships and interactions that are part of daily life.*

# *Personal Triumph*

## Jerry McNeight

OREGON

Jerry McNeight from chapter 7 admits that he likes doing things on his own and living life his way. He never imagined himself joining Weight Watchers. Jerry, a trucking analyst and outdoor enthusiast, enjoys being athletic.

"I like challenges. I have done some crazy things in my life. At one point, I decided to take up mountain climbing. I climbed a lot of mountains, even Mount Everest. My doctors told me that mountain climbing would destroy my knees and hips, and it did. So I got new knees and hips and spent a lot of time sitting home alone feeling sorry for myself. I couldn't do a lot of things anymore and I got big. I blamed it on my knees; my doctor blamed it on my weight and told me to join Weight Watchers. I prefer doing things alone and on my terms."

*"Believe me, although I've changed some of my habits, I still do things my way."*

Jerry tried to lose weight. He dropped a lot of pounds using an extreme method, but then gained them all back. He tried taking pills that promised to take off pounds while he slept; they did nothing.

"One day, a bunch of women in my office joined a Weight Watchers At Work Meeting. They dared me to start with them. I knew that they would goad me and pester me until I joined, so I did. I got on a roll and lost 80 pounds to my goal. Believe me, although I've changed some of my habits, I still do things my way."

Jerry now goes on 100-mile bicycle rides every other weekend.

## You and Your Partner

The person you live with affects your weight and your weight affects that person. As we've discussed, part of your weight is determined by your genes, so you are more likely to be overweight if one or both of your parents were heavy. While genetics do play a role, so does living together. Weight patterns and the likelihood of overweight run together in spouses and partners and also in households of other people who are living together but do not share a blood link.

In studies looking at men and women during their first year of marriage, weight gain is common for both partners. As Dr. Rippe experienced when he got married, this pattern of weight gain with marriage, especially for men, is so universal that a paper from the Centers for Disease Control and Prevention recommended that an effective public health strategy to prevent weight gain may be to counsel men about the risks of marriage!

The togetherness of weight lasts beyond the first year of marriage. The connection between the weights of spouses seems to last for as long as the marriage does. Not surprisingly, the reason spouses seem to have similar weight classifications—healthy or overweight—is at least partly due to their shared environment. Living together, talking together, eating together, and sharing leisure time certainly affects weight in both direct and indirect ways. Studies done on the weight/marriage connection indicate that the effects may be due to the influence of eating meals together, a shared commitment or lack of commitment to controlling weight, or both. Regardless, the decision to lose weight has an impact on both your ability to lose weight and the environment you share with your partner.

Because the life you share with a partner is so linked with everything that you do, it makes sense that spouses and partners who decide to lose weight at the same time have better success. Weight-loss programs that include couples find that the weight loss of each member of the couple is significantly better at the end of the program and for several months afterward when compared to the people who attend the same kind of weight-loss program alone. It seems that couple-attended programs provide a different kind or quality of social support.

Certainly the benefits of losing weight as a couple are clear. But there may be less direct benefits to the partner who is not actively attending a weight-loss program, especially if this person is a husband. The husbands of the women participating in the reduced-fat diet section of the Women's Health Trial lost more weight over three years than the spouses of women in the control group. While the absolute weight loss was not large, it is interesting because the men were unknowingly eating less butter, margarine, eggs, and red meat. And the more meals the couple shared, the bigger the effect. So even if you think you are changing your eating patterns and food choices as a lone effort, you may be helping your mate.

While it helps weight-loss success if you can do it as a team with a spouse or partner, it is not a requirement. In a study that looked at this specific aspect of weight loss, marriages that had moderate levels of friction were not an insurmountable barrier to successful weight loss. When it comes to marriage and weight loss, your partner can be a big help, but he or she does not need to be an obstacle to your achieving your goals.

## You and Your Family

Just as weight is one piece of the pie that defines the relationship you have with your partner, it is also a component of the relationships you have with other family members, especially your children. The weight-related attitudes and behavior of mothers influence the way their children, especially their daughters, view their body shape. For example, the value a child places on a slim body is affected by the size of her family, with heavier families tending to have children putting greater significance on this personal attribute than children whose families are at a healthy weight. Furthermore, parents' eating habits strongly influence the eating habits of other family members. This is true before the decision to lose weight happens, while weight is being lost, and during sustained weight loss.

# Personal Triumph

## Katherine Deliso

MASSACHUSETTS

*"I helped my parents to understand portions and my new way of eating."*

Katherine Deliso, the librarian we were introduced to in chapter 8, had to work closely with her parents after she joined Weight Watchers. "I live with my parents. My first couple of weeks on Weight Watchers were difficult because I wanted everyone around me to follow the Weight Watchers program.

"I helped my parents to understand portions and my new way of eating. They are very supportive now. My father always asks me which foods I'd like to have. He now tells friends that I have lost weight and that he is proud of my success."

Katherine dropped five dress sizes in reaching her goal.

Parents set the stage for positive and negative eating behaviors within the household. Children with overweight parents have been found to have a higher preference for high-fat foods, a lower preference for vegetables, and a more indulgent eating style. They are also more sedentary. Conversely, having fruits and vegetables in the house and parents who eat them has the children eating them too. Let's take a more detailed look at how the different roles parents play affect their children.

*Parents are providers.* Food served at home, especially in the early years, sets the stage for a child's future eating behaviors. Children are influenced by positive actions. Young children of parents who keep plenty of fruits and vegetables in the house are more likely to eat fruits and vegetables during their school-age years. In contrast, children who prefer high-fat, high-sugar foods over other foods seem to develop this preference in homes where these foods are available in abundance and are routinely eaten by other family members. That does not mean that banning these types of foods from the house is a good idea, however.

Interestingly, children whose parents are inconsistent in having high-fat, high-sugar foods in the house also learn to prefer these foods. If there is a history of sporadically following extreme diets in the house and if periods of no treats in the house are followed by lots of treats in the house, a child is more likely to develop a preference for junk foods and overeat them when they are available.

*Parents are enforcers.* How a parent enforces food rules affects a child's eating habits. Several studies show that pushing a particular food on children increases the likelihood of the child developing a dislike for it. Children who will not eat fruits and vegetables were often encouraged or even forced to eat them when they were younger. The opposite is also true: restricting foods actually causes children to eat more of them, more often. Many parents don't know this. In a 1989 study published in the journal *Appetite,* 40% of parents said that restricting or forbidding a particular food would teach their child not to like it. In fact, several studies have shown that forbidding a food actually increases the child's preference for and intake of that food. Parents who play the role of food police do more harm than good.

*Parents are role models*. Most importantly, a parent's eating behavior and attitudes strongly affect a child's eating. Children watch and learn from their parents and mimic parental behaviors. Women who chronically follow highly restrictive diets have daughters who tend to do so as well. Both mothers and fathers who have high levels of food disinhibition have daughters with the same disinhibition. Parental role models affect a child's activity level as well. Children of parents who are physically active and encourage family activities are more likely to become physically active.

By breaking through the myths of weight loss yourself, you have the opportunity to share your experience with your family. By achieving a lasting weight loss with a comprehensive program that includes eating in a style that demonstrates flexible restraint, being physically active, and maintaining a positive mindset, you will create a home that supports a healthy weight for everyone who lives there.

Just as your weight loss affects the people you live with, those you live with can have a big impact on weight-loss success. A supportive family is a tremendous boost to weight-loss efforts. In one study involving Mexican-American adults enrolled in a lifestyle-based weight-loss program, those who involved their families lost the most weight.

### You and the World

The impact of weight extends beyond the family. Friends and coworkers also affect your weight-loss success. One of the Institute of Medicine (IOM) factors for weight-loss success is attending a weight-loss program. We also know that losing weight as a couple is effective. This strategy of teamwork extends to friends as well. In a study conducted in Pittsburgh, it was found that people who joined a weight-loss program with friends lost more weight and sustained the weight loss better than those who joined the program alone. Getting knowledge and encouragement from a weight-loss program that is reinforced by friends creates the supportive atmosphere that is important to achieving weight loss that lasts.

# *Personal Triumph*

## Jenny Hennessey

CONNECTICUT

Jenny Hennessey, an accountant, always thought that she could lose weight on her own. She watched her weight go up and down her entire life—whenever she lost, she went back to her old ways and gained it back. Around Christmas one year, Jenny saw some photos of herself in a ball gown. She didn't like what she saw.

> *"My children have been so supportive of me. They don't push me to eat foods I don't want, and they accept my personal food choices without asking questions."*

Around the same time, a neighbor mentioned that a few friends were joining Weight Watchers and invited her to come along. Jenny joined. She loves the program's flexibility because she and her family can eat the same foods at meals.

"My children have been so supportive of me. They don't push me to eat foods I don't want, and they accept my personal food choices."

Although it would be wonderful if you could count on universal encouragement from everybody around you when it comes to your weight loss, this may not be the case. It is not uncommon to have family members and friends who consciously or unconsciously sabotage your weight-loss efforts. A friend may be jealous of your success. A spouse or partner may make negative comments or push food because he or she is afraid of rejection once his or her spouse or partner gets slim. Friends who were eating or drinking buddies may not understand your desire to make the choices that are part of successful weight loss, so they may try to persuade you to indulge in your old favorites. A successful approach to weight loss must include strategies for dealing with food pressures or a lack of encouragement from others. Learning from the experiences of others who have successfully overcome these kinds of challenges can be particularly helpful.

### You Can Even Enlist the IRS to Help You

With all the negative health issues that come with overweight, it is not surprising that health care costs go up with weight. Studies have shown that, insurance aside, people who are overweight pay 11.4% more for health care out-of-pocket expenses, and as weight increases, that number goes up.

The good news is that the Internal Revenue Service has ruled that the costs for qualified weight-loss programs (including programs such as Weight Watchers) may be considered a medical deduction. That means that if your physician prescribes the program, you can include the relevant costs as tax deductions for medical care. Alternatively, you can use your employer-sponsored medical savings account or flexible savings account to pay for qualified weight-loss services with tax-exempt dollars. Certain qualifications apply, so be sure to check with your tax professional. More information is available at the Web site for the American Obesity Association: www.obesity.org.

## The Bottom Line

While it is true that weight is a highly personal issue and individual commitment is a key to success, it is not a one-person issue. It affects family, friends, and those around you in both direct and indirect ways. The positive changes that lead to sustainable weight loss—a positive mindset, wise food choices, regular physical activity, and a supportive atmosphere—benefit those close to you.

# *Personal Triumph*

## Jenny Hennessey

CONNECTICUT

In addition to strong family support, Jenny Hennessey wanted the strong support of a Meeting Leader. After some missteps, Jenny settled into a meeting that had a Leader with whom she felt a rapport.

"My Leader was such a great coach. She pointed out to me why I was not losing weight and gave me some great suggestions. Guess what? I had a great weight loss during the first week that I tried her advice. I attribute so much of my success to the coaching and the support at my meeting.

"I feel accountable to my Meeting Leader. She inspires and motivates me because she talks from experience. She is a great coach, always telling me that I can stick with my new habits and that I'm going to make it. I also feel responsible to other people who are trying to lose weight. They can learn from what I went through."

*"I attribute so much of my success to the coaching from my Leader and the support at my meeting."*

Jenny lost about 35 pounds to reach her goal.

## Weight Loss That Lasts

# Action Steps

Weight loss does not have to be a solo event. There are benefits to be gained and benefits that can be shared with the people you care about.

- Consider opening up to the people around you. Explain to them how important losing weight is for you and be specific about how they can best help you.
- Create your team to lose weight. Team up with people with whom you feel comfortable and who you are confident will encourage your efforts.
- Live in a healthy weight home. Be a role model to your spouse and your children. By following the lifestyle habits that will lead you to sustained weight loss, you'll be influencing their food and exercise behaviors as well.
- Recognize and celebrate the health-related changes in the quality of life that come with weight loss!

# Conclusion

## Your personal triumph

Weight loss is fraught with myths, and we've delved into ten of the most common ones in this book. Like any myth, each of the weight-loss myths we have explored has kernels of truth. But a kernel of truth is not the whole truth, and it is only by gaining knowledge about the whole truth that sustained weight loss is possible.

## Truths Instead of Myths

Let's recap the fundamental truths behind each of the ten myths in this book to get you thinking about all that you have learned and how you can use this knowledge to create your own weight-loss success story.

### 1. Sustained weight loss *is* possible.

Despite a lot of belief to the contrary, millions of people have achieved lasting weight loss. The factors linked with both successful weight loss and lasting weight loss have been identified. Databases of thousands of people who have achieved and are maintaining a healthy body weight have been established, and they are fascinating and instructive. The key factors include setting realistic goals and actively participating in a comprehensive weight-loss program that includes a nutritious way of eating, attention to exercise, changing behaviors and thinking patterns to those that support a healthy weight, and being surrounded by a supportive atmosphere.

### 2. Weight is a health issue.

Extensive research has shown that Body Mass Index (BMI) provides a good estimate of body fat and is directly linked with health. As BMI goes up from 25, the risk of developing coronary heart disease, high cholesterol, hypertension, diabetes, metabolic syndrome (Syndrome X), and several forms of cancer also goes up. The higher the BMI, the higher the risk, especially if body fat tends to accumulate at the waist. While health deteriorates with excess weight, it improves quickly and significantly with weight loss. Losing 5% to 10% of body weight has a positive influence on health, enhancing body's use of insulin, lowering blood pressure, decreasing triglyceride levels, and improving cholesterol values. A greater weight loss brings even more health benefits.

### 3. Willpower is only a small piece of what is needed to achieve weight loss that lasts.

It is not possible to will something to happen if the stage is not properly set up. For weight loss, that means being knowledgeable about what you need in a comprehensive program, choosing a method that provides you with the essential elements, and developing skills and strategies that make the method work within the context of your daily life.

### 4. Exercise is not an effective, stand-alone weight-loss method.

Increasing activity without making changes in eating is unlikely to produce weight loss. Exercise is, however, a critical component of a comprehensive weight-loss program along with attention to food choices, having a positive mindset, and creating a supportive atmosphere. There are many health benefits to exercise, and its role in keeping weight off is well established. The best way to increase metabolism and burn more calories is to enjoy regular physical activity that burns calories and builds muscle.

### 5. Cutting calories, not avoiding fats or carbohydrates, is at the heart of weight loss.

A diet that provides the right mix of macronutrients is best for losing weight because it provides the variety needed in an eating pattern that can be sustained. Foods that are rich sources of fats or carbohydrates provide essential nutrients for good health, but not all fats or carbohydrates are created equal with their impact on health. It's important to be knowledgeable about making wise food choices that promote weight loss and health.

### 6. Sustainable weight loss is possible *for you*.

While we are all individuals with our own set of genes, metabolism, and body type, the basic principles of what it takes to achieve lasting weight loss are the same. Some people have a genetic or a personal profile that makes them more vulnerable to weight gain, but that does not mean weight loss is impossible. Biology is not destiny. Being knowledgeable about the factors that affect weight can be helpful in setting realistic expectations about weight loss and selecting approaches that are most likely to be helpful to you.

### 7. The only way to lose weight is to take in fewer calories or burn more calories than the body needs.

That means eating fewer calories and becoming more physically active. The key to successful weight loss is to invest your time and energy in establishing the behaviors that make this happen. It is counterproductive to spend time and effort on things that do not make a difference, such as eating specific combinations of food, focusing on meal timing, and taking pills and supplements, to name a few.

### 8. The method you choose for your weight loss matters a great deal.

A method that leads to lasting weight-loss success paces the rate of weight loss, avoiding extreme lifestyle changes that are unlikely to be sustained. Take progressive steps in implementing change over time.

Following a method that does all of these things creates a smooth transition from losing weight to keeping the weight off.

**9. There is no single right approach to weight loss.**

Science has shown us what is needed to achieve sustained weight loss. A comprehensive weight-loss program takes those elements and converts them into a method or guidelines that will result in the desired outcome. But you need to individualize the approach—the skills, strategies, and approaches—of how the method is followed. Every person has preferences, habits, priorities, and a lifestyle that are uniquely her or his own. Achieving weight loss that lasts requires following a comprehensive weight-loss program in a way that works for you.

**10. While losing weight is a personal issue, it affects other people and can be helped or hurt by the people around you.**

Each person's weight is a part of who they are, regardless of the number of pounds on the scale. Weight impacts the individual's quality of life as well as relationships with partners, family, and friends. It follows that whenever there is a change in weight, there is an impact on everyone. Sustained weight loss has a very positive impact on people you care about. One of the pillars of a comprehensive weight-loss program is developing and living in a supportive atmosphere. People around you can help you reach your goals.

## Use Your Knowledge

This book has provided you with the knowledge you need to break through the myths that may have been holding you back in the past. By learning about and understanding the abundance of science that surrounds sustained weight loss, you are now in the perfect position to make informed choices.

You know that when it comes to weight loss that lasts, you need a comprehensive weight-loss program. That program needs to have four pillars: food, exercise, behavior, and a supportive atmosphere. The program needs to be flexible, healthy, realistic, sustainable, and livable. No single approach works for everyone, so you need to seek out the tips, strategies, and approaches that will work for you. Then you need to start them, practice them, refine them, and make them your own.

It is now up to you to put your knowledge into action. Enjoy the ride!

# Afterword

## A personal message from Karen Miller-Kovach, Chief Scientific Officer, Weight Watchers International

Weight Watchers decided to write this book with Dr. Jim Rippe because as an organization we are committed to providing a comprehensive weight-loss program based on the latest scientific thinking. All too often in weight loss, a program or product is developed and then individual studies that support the program are provided to justify its existence. This approach of pick-and-choose science at least in part explains how weight-loss myths get started and then make their way into the lore that surrounds weight loss.

Weight Watchers is committed to providing a weight-loss program that comes out of the science, not the other way around. This book is intended to take you behind the curtain of science and give you the knowledge you need to put yourself on the path of sustained weight loss. By knowing which myths are holding you back and gaining the knowledge to break through them, you will be able to achieve weight loss that lasts.

But knowing and doing are often two different things. It is not unusual for a person to walk into Weight Watchers and say, "I am committed to losing weight and know that I want to do it in a healthy, effective way. I know that losing weight is about calories, making different food choices, and being more physically active. I am also concerned about my health and I want to maximize the health benefits that come with weight loss, so I know that I need to have a balanced diet and do the right amount and kinds of exercise. I know all that—but what do I eat for lunch?"

These people come to Weight Watchers because our program teaches them a method to help them put that knowledge into practice. For those who may be unfamiliar with the Weight Watchers method, here is a look at our program and how we take the science that is presented in this book and turn it into a program that is helping millions of people around the world achieve weight loss that lasts.

## The Bird's-Eye View

Throughout its history of more than forty years, the Weight Watchers program has been built on a consistent foundation. There are four principles from which Weight Watchers will not waver:

1. Any program developed by Weight Watchers must provide healthy weight loss. This principle translates into a program designed to

   - Produce a rate of weight loss of up to 2 pounds per week after the first three weeks when losses may be greater due to water loss.
   - Guide food choices that not only reduce calories but meet current scientific recommendations for nutritional completeness and reduced disease risk.
   - Construct an activity plan that provides the full range of weight- and health-related benefits that exercise offers.

- Be sustainable—healthy weight loss *is* weight loss that lasts, so the program must go beyond losing the excess weight and address keeping it off.

2. In addition to being healthy, any Weight Watchers program must be realistic, practical, and livable. It must also be flexible enough so that people can apply the approaches that work well for them. That means encouraging the achievement of realistic goals. For example, we do not recommend that a person with a lot of weight to lose begin the program with a weight-loss goal that defines ultimate success. Rather, we start with our *10% goal,* or losing 10% of body weight (for example, a 10% goal for someone who is 200 pounds is 20 pounds). As you've learned from this book, a weight loss of 10% translates into significant health benefits. We believe this should be recognized and the achievement of this goal should be celebrated, so we have built this into the program and focus on the selection and celebration of interim goals as part of the weight-loss process.

   Likewise, pacing weight loss and following a system that encourages food and activity choices that are livable and sustainable in the real world is key. The Weight Watchers program is designed on the premise that weight management needs to *fit into* your life, not *be* your life. That translates into providing a method that enables you to develop the skill of flexible restraint so important to sustained weight loss.

3. Weight Watchers believes in imparting knowledge. Rather than creating an aura of mysticism around its program, Weight Watchers believes that people should learn not only what to do but why. This knowledge brings understanding, and with understanding comes the confidence needed to make informed choices and live by them.

4. Finally, every program provided by Weight Watchers must be comprehensive. As you have learned in this book, sustained

weight loss comes from taking a holistic view of all its components: food, activity, behavior, and a supportive atmosphere. Now let's take a look at how each of those pillars gets translated into a science-based program.

## Food

It is often said that different paths can lead to the same destination, and nowhere is that more true than eating for healthy weight loss. Each person is unique when it comes to foods that provide eating satisfaction, preferred meals and times of day to eat, and the style of making food choices for sustained weight loss. Weight-loss success depends on finding a method that fits within one's lifestyle and preferences. The Weight Watchers food plans are designed to make this happen.

Through our research we have found that there are two distinct approaches to controlling calories. One is based on tracking and controlling how much you eat. The other approach is based on focusing on a group of wholesome foods without counting or tracking. The Weight Watchers TurnAround™ program offers two different food plans based on these two distinct approaches to eating for lasting weight loss. People can use these two approaches to structure their eating in a way that fits their life. We have found that the best way to lose weight is for a person to pick the approach that makes sense for him or her. Here is a snapshot of the two plans and the approaches:

1. The **Flex Plan** is based on the Weight Watchers patented ***POINTS***® Food System. This approach is designed to allow you to eat any food as long as you keep track and control how much you eat. Every food has a ***POINTS*** value—a small, easy-to-remember number (for example, 1, 2, 3). The number is based on the calories, grams of total fat, and grams of dietary fiber for a specific portion of the food. The system does not require exact weighing and measuring but instead encourages people to focus on the bigger picture by building awareness of the food choices

they make and eating reasonable portions. The ***POINTS*** formula gently guides food choices by encouraging the selection of healthy foods with a lower energy density because that's where you get the most food for a given ***POINTS*** value. Based on a person's current weight, a ***POINTS*** Target is established—the total of ***POINTS*** values for the day. Choosing foods to meet the target ensures a healthful rate of weight loss. On the Flex Plan, tracking and controlling your food intake allows you to lose weight while having the entire variety of foods available.

2. The **Core Plan** controls calories by focusing eating on a core list of wholesome nutritious foods without counting. The list is comprised of foods from all the food groups: fruits and vegetables; grains and starches; lean meats, fish, and poultry; eggs; and dairy products. We preselected these foods to provide eating satisfaction without empty calories. They are low in energy density and have a low potential for overeating based on our research. For the occasional treat, you can also eat foods outside of this list in a controlled amount. This approach allows you to eat healthfully and lose weight without counting or tracking.

As you learned from this book, developing the skill of flexible restraint when it comes to eating is important for weight-loss success. To help build this skill, both the Flex Plan and the Core Plan include a feature called the Weekly Allowance. The Weekly Allowance provides a system for having treats and indulgences without sacrificing weight loss. By using this feature and experiencing the ability to incorporate day-to-day food challenges into a method that provides weight loss without rigid food rules, the invaluable skill of flexible restraint is learned.

On both plans, people eat real food they can buy at any grocery store or order when dining out. The program does not require buying and eating any specific foods. This makes weight management easier, more livable, and more enjoyable.

Whatever approach is used, some fundamental food choices are essential for good health and nutrition. The Weight Watchers program covers these in its Healthy Eating Guidelines, which recommends that every day you

- Include at least five servings of fruits and vegetables
- Have at least two servings of milk; three if you are a teen or over 50 years old
- Drink at least six glasses of water
- Get a serving or two of a protein-rich food
- Take a multiple vitamin-mineral supplement
- Limit added sugars and alcohol
- Have some healthy oil, like olive, canola, sunflower, safflower, or flaxseed
- Choose whole-grain foods whenever possible

Finding an eating approach that works is key to weight-loss success. The Weight Watchers food plans are designed to reach the objective of a healthy weight loss, but they do so by empowering the person to make food choices in a way that suits his or her preferences and lifestyle. We believe this is the only way that sustained weight loss is feasible.

## Exercise

The Weight Watchers program provides a systematic approach to exercise throughout the weight-loss process. Research shows that beginning a structured food and exercise program at the same time is not as successful as beginning them at separate times. Therefore, the Weight Watchers program starts with focusing on the food plan, then brings the specifics of activity into the method a couple of weeks later once people have had a chance to master their eating plan. That does not mean that the role of activity in a comprehensive weight-loss program is not addressed from the beginning. Rather, while a person is getting started on learning the mechanics of a food plan, we recommend that activity changes focus on reducing sedentary behavior. Rather than meeting specific activity targets, the focus is to spend less time sitting. Taking the stairs instead of the elevator, parking at the far end of a parking lot, or making a walk a part of daily life does not require a great deal of effort, is doable, and does not reduce the focus on learning a food plan.

After a couple of weeks of reducing sedentary behavior, the ***POINTS*** Activity System is introduced. In a way that complements the ***POINTS*** values of food, a formula that calculates the ***POINTS*** values for activity is used. The formula is based on body weight, the amount of time the activity is done, and the level of intensity. This method enables a person to do any exercise or activity that is enjoyable and fits within his or her lifestyle. It provides a flexible approach to activity that is accurate in its estimation of the calories burned because it is based on the individual.

As you have learned from this book, the recommended amounts of activity vary based on the desired goal of doing the exercise. Getting the health benefits of exercise takes less time and effort than the amount recommended for weight loss. The amount of activity associated with maintaining a weight goal is even more. For this reason, the Weight Watchers program adjusts the recommended ***POINTS*** Target for activity as weight loss proceeds, beginning with the amount needed to gain health benefits and progressing so that the recommended amount of activity for sustained weight loss is met at the time that the ultimate weight goal is achieved.

One added feature of the ***POINTS*** Weight-Loss System is that ***POINTS*** values earned in activity can be swapped for additional food on a one-to-one basis.

## Behavior

Making changes in behavior is at the heart of sustained weight loss, but it doesn't just happen. Two specific components of behavior change are keys to the Weight Watchers program: self-monitoring and cognitive skills—cognitive is a scientific term that means how you think.

We cover the science of self-monitoring as part of sustainable weight loss in this book. There are two important pieces to self-monitoring—having a way to maintain awareness about what is being done and including a method to assess weight-loss progress. The Weight Watchers program includes both.

Monitoring eating behavior on the Weight Watchers program differs for each food plan. Because the Flex Plan requires tracking ***POINTS*** values to reach the daily ***POINTS*** Target, we developed the QuikTrak™ System. This system includes a flexible, easy-to-use journal where the specific food choices can be recorded, or, if desired, a simple check-off method to count down the ***POINTS*** values as they are used. The Core Plan does not require counting ***POINTS*** values but rather focuses on eating as much as is needed to feel satisfied from a core list of wholesome, nutritious foods. The self-monitoring method for the Core Plan involves using a Comfort Zone scale to assess hunger and fullness on an ongoing basis. While the approaches are different, both the Flex Plan and the Core Plan include self-monitoring to keep awareness of food choices high—a key component to sustained weight loss.

To monitor weight-loss progress, the weekly weigh-in is a fundamental part of the Weight Watchers program. The weigh-in is confidential and done by a trained Weight Watchers staff member. Weight information is never shared outside the weigh-in. Many people find the accountability of being weighed by another person helpful to their weight-loss efforts and the structure of going to a Weight Watchers meeting each week a way to keep their commitment high. Weight Watchers recommends that weight be taken only once a week during the weight-loss process, preferably in a consistent way (as to the time of day or day of the week) to avoid putting too much emphasis on the erratic scale as a measure of progress.

Regular weighing is also a key factor in sustained weight loss. Weight Watchers has a unique system to encourage this behavior for people who have reached their weight goal on the program. Any Weight Watchers member who reaches a healthy body weight (defined as a Body Mass Index between 20 and 25 or a weight goal prescribed by a qualified health professional) and successfully completes the six-week weight maintenance phase of the program becomes a Lifetime Member (LTM) of Weight Watchers. In this book you've read the personal triumphs of many LTMs and learned about some of the methods they use to keep the weight off.

LTMs are asked to weigh in once a month at a Weight Watchers meeting. When an LTM weighs in within 2 pounds of his or her goal weight, he or she can attend Weight Watchers meetings anywhere in the world at no cost for that month. This unique system allows Weight Watchers to provide its members two of the elements that predict sustained weight loss in the Institute of Medicine (IOM) report: monitoring weight and continued contact with those who were part of the weight-loss process.

In addition to monitoring, the Program teaches a series of specific techniques that enhance cognitive behavior, or thinking skills: the Weight Watchers Tools for Living. These techniques are proven strategies that restructure internal thought processes in a way that enhances the ability to make long-term positive changes. The techniques include tools like Motivating Strategy and Storyboarding, and they enable a person to interact and thrive in the weight-challenging situations and social interactions that make up daily life.

## A Supportive Atmosphere

Learning to create and live in a supportive atmosphere that aids weight loss is a defining aspect of the Weight Watchers experience. As a member of Weight Watchers, a person attends a weekly meeting. The meetings are conducted by a Weight Watchers Leader. All of the Leaders are successful members who have become LTMs and have also undergone extensive training that includes mastering the specifics of the Weight Watchers program, guiding people in making positive changes in their lives, and facilitating meetings. Because all of the Leaders have achieved sustained weight loss on the Weight Watchers program, they are role models and a source of inspiration and information.

The Weight Watchers meeting includes people who are at different stages of their weight loss, including LTMs who have weighed in and are attending the meeting for free. They are a source of practical tips and experiences that members can benefit from for their own weight management. Each Weight Watchers meeting includes the confidential weigh-in to monitor weight-loss progress, information about the Weight Watchers program, and a discussion of a new topic related to nutrition, activity, and healthy habits. In addition to the meeting, more information and communication with other members is found at any hour of the day or night on WeightWatchers.com.

Many people who have achieved sustained weight loss with Weight Watchers tell us they believe attending the meetings was the single biggest reason they were successful.

## The Bottom, Bottom Line

The Weight Watchers program is built on a strong foundation of science. Throughout this book, we have shared the findings and conclusions that define the science of sustained weight loss.

Four of the most influential and knowledgeable organizations when it comes to weight and health issues—the World Health Organization, the National Institutes of Health, the U.S. Surgeon General's Office, and the Institute of Medicine—have convened panels of experts to evaluate the pool of science and condense it into reports of what works. The Weight Watchers program has embraced these reports. We have taken these expert-derived scientific documents and conducted extensive research of our own to put them into an easy-to-learn and simple-to-follow weight-loss method.

Our goal is to provide a program based on science as well as one that lives in the real world, and our program is followed by millions of people with great success.

# Sources

## List of Abbreviations

| | |
|---|---|
| Addict Behav | Addictive Behaviors |
| Am J Clin Nutr | American Journal of Clinical Nutrition |
| Am J Epidemiol | American Journal of Epidemiology |
| Am J Health Behav | American Journal of Health Behavior |
| Am J Med | American Journal of Medicine |
| Am J Prev Med | American Journal of Preventive Medicine |
| Am J Public Health | American Journal of Public Health |
| Am Psychol | The American Psychologist |
| Ann Behav Med | Annals of Behavioral Medicine |
| Ann Intern Med | Annals of Internal Medicine |
| Ann Nutr Metab | Annals of Nutrition & Metabolism |
| Annu Rev Nutr | Annual Review of Nutrition |
| Appetite | Appetite |
| Arch Intern Med | Archives of Internal Medicine |
| Arq Bras Cardiol | Arquivos Brasileiros de Cardiologia |
| Asia Pac J Clin Nutr | Asia-Pacific Journal of Clinical Nutrition |
| Behav Processes | Behavioural Processes |
| Br J Nutr | The British Journal of Nutrition |
| Cancer | Cancer |
| Chronobiol Int | Chronobiology International |
| Circulation | Circulation |
| Climacteric | Climacteric |
| Clin Cornerstone | Clinical Cornerstone |
| Crit Rev Food Sci Nutr | CRC Critical Reviews in Food Science and Nutrition |
| Curr Atheroscler Rep | Current Atherosclerosis Reports |
| Diabetes Care | Diabetes Care |
| Diabetes Nutr Metab | Diabetes, Nutrition & Metabolism |
| Dis Colon Rectum | Diseases of the Colon and Rectum |
| Eat Behav | Eating Behaviors |

| | |
|---|---|
| Eat Weight Disord | Eating and Weight Disorders |
| Endocrinol Metab Clin North Am | Endocrinology and Metabolism Clinics of North America |
| Ethn Dis | Ethnicity & Disease |
| FDA Consumer | FDA Consumer |
| Health Affairs | Health Affairs |
| Health Educ Behav | Health Education & Behavior |
| Health Psychol | Health Psychology |
| Int J Eat Disord | International Journal of Eating Disorders |
| Int J Obes Relat Metab Disord | International Journal of Obesity and Related Metabolic Disorders |
| Int J Sport Nutr | International Journal of Sports Nutrition |
| J Aging Health | Journal of Aging and Health |
| JAMA | Journal of the American Medical Association |
| J Am Coll Cardiol | Journal of the American College of Cardiology |
| J Am Coll Nutr | Journal of the American College of Nutrition |
| J Am Diet Assoc | Journal of the American Dietetic Association |
| J Am Soc Nephrol | Journal of the American Society of Nephrology |
| J Appl Psychol | Journal of Applied Psychology |
| J Behav Ther Exp Psychiatry | Journal of Behavior Therapy and Experimental Psychiatry |
| J Cardiopulm Rehab | Journal of Cardiopulmonary Rehabilitation |
| J Consult Clin Psychol | Journal of Consulting and Clinical Psychology |
| J Women's Health (Larchmnt) | Journal of Women's Health |
| Mech Ageing Dev | Mechanisms of Ageing and Development |
| Med J Aust | The Medical Journal of Australia |
| Med Sci Sports Exerc | Medicine and Science in Sports and Exercise |
| MMWR Morb Mortal Wkly Rep | MMWR: Morbidity and Mortality Weekly Report |
| N Engl J Med | New England Journal of Medicine |
| Nutrition | Nutrition |
| Nutr Metab Cardiovasc Dis | Nutrition, Metabolism, and Cardiovascular Diseases |
| Nutr Rev | Nutrition Reviews |
| Obes Res | Obesity Research |
| Obes Rev | Obesity Reviews |
| Obes Surg | Obesity Surgery |
| Obstet Gyn | Obstetrics and Gynecology |
| Pediatrics | Pediatrics |
| Physiol Behav | Physiology & Behavior |
| Proc Nutr Soc | The Proceedings of the Nutrition Society |
| Public Health Nutr | Public Health Nutrition |
| Rev Med Liege | Revue Medicale de Liege |
| Sci Aging Knowledge Environ | Science of Aging Knowledge Environment |
| Soc Sci Med | Social Science & Medicine |
| West Indian Med J | The West Indian Medical Journal |

## Chapter 1: Is sustainable weight loss possible?

Brownell KD. The central role of lifestyle change in long-term weight management. *Clin Cornerstone* 1999;2:43–51.

Brownell KD, Rodin J. The dieting maelstrom. Is it possible and advisable to lose weight? *Am Psychol* 1994;49:781–91.

Foster GD, Wadden TA, Phelan S, Sarwer DB, Sanderson RS. Obese patients' perceptions of treatment outcomes and the factors that influence them. *Arch Intern Med* 2001;161:2133–9.

Heshka S, Anderson JW, Atkinson RL, Greenaway FL, Hill JO, Phinney SD, Kolotkin RL, Miller-Kovach K, PiSunyer FX. Weight loss with self-help compared with a structured commercial program: a randomized trial. *JAMA* 2003;289:1792–8.

Institute of Medicine. *Weighing the Options. Criteria for Evaluating Weight-Management Programs*. Washington, DC: National Academy Press, 1995.

Lowe MR, Thaw J, Miller-Kovach K. Long-term follow-up assessment of successful dieters in a commercial weight-loss program. *Int J Obes Relat Metab Disord* 2004;28(suppl 1):S29.

McGuire MT, Wing RR, Hill JO. The prevalence of weight loss maintenance among American adults. *Int J Obes Relat Metab Disord* 1999;23:1314–9.

*Methods for Voluntary Weight Loss and Control*. Technol Assess Conf Statement; 1992 Mar 30–Apr 1. Bethesda, MD: National Institutes of Health, Office of Medical Applications of Research; 1992.

National Heart, Lung, and Blood Institute. *Clinical Guidelines on the Identification, Evaluation, and Treatment of Overweight and Obesity in Adults*. NIH Publication No. 98-4083. Bethesda, MD: National Institutes of Health, September 1998.

National Heart, Lung, and Blood Institute. *The Practical Guide. Identification, Evaluation, and Treatment of Overweight and Obesity in Adults*. NIH Publication No. 00-4084. Bethesda, MD: National Institutes of Health, October 2000.

Weinsier RL, Nagy TR, Hunter GR, Darnell BE, Hensrud DD, Weiss HL. Do adaptive changes in metabolic rate favor weight regain in weight-reduced individuals? An examination of the set-point theory. *Am J Clin Nutr* 2000;72:1088–94.

Wing RR, Hill JO. Successful weight loss maintenance. *Annu Rev Nutr* 2001;21:323–41.

## Chapter 2: Do those extra few pounds really matter?

American College of Sports Medicine. www.acsm.org/pdf/bonemscl.pdf.

American Heart Association. *Heart Disease and Stroke Statistics—2004 Update*. Dallas, TX: American Heart Association, 2003.

American Obesity Society. www.obesity.org.

Ballard-Barbash R. Anthropometry and breast cancer. Body size—a moving target. *Cancer* 1994;74(suppl 3):1090–1100.

Calle EE, Thun MJ, Petrelli JM, Rodriguez C, Heath CW. Body mass index and mortality in a prospective cohort of U.S. adults. *N Engl J Med* 1999;341:1097–1105.

Chan JM, Rimm EB, Colditz GA, et al. Obesity, fat distribution, and weight gain as risk factors for clinical diabetes in men. *Diabetes Care* 1994;17:961–9.

Colditz GA, Willett WC, Rotnitzky A, Manson JE. Weight gain as a risk factor for clinical diabetes mellitus in women. *Ann Intern Med* 1995;122:481–6.

Colditz GA, Willett WC, Stampfer MJ, et al. Weight as a risk factor for clinical diabetes in women. *Am J Epidemiol* 1990;132:501–13.

Dobs MS. Effects of testerosterone on body composition of the aging male. *Mech Ageing Dev* 2004;125:297–304.

Feigelson, H. *Cancer Epidemiology, Biomarkers & Prevention*. February 2004;13:220–4. News release, American Cancer Society.

Ford ES, Williamson DF, Liu S. Weight change and diabetes incidence: findings from a national cohort of US adults. *Am J Epidemiol* 1997;146:214–22.

Jenkins KR. Body-weight change and physical functioning among young old adults. J *Aging Health* 2004;16:248–66.

Kyle UG, Morabia A, Schutz Y, Pichard C. Sedentarism affects body fat mass index and fat-free mass index in adults aged 18 to 98 years. *Nutrition* 2004;20:255–60.

Milewicz A, Tworowska U, Demissie M. Menopausal obesity—myth or fact? *Climacteric* 2001;4:273–83.

Mizuno T, Shu IW, Makimura H, Mobbs C. Obesity over the life course. *Sci Aging Knowledge Environ* 2004;June 16 (24):RE4.

Molitch ME, Fujimoto W, Hamman RF, Knowler WC. Diabetes Prevention Program Research Group. The diabetes prevention program and its global implications. *J Am Soc Nephrol* 2003;147(suppl 2):S103–7.

National Heart, Lung, and Blood Institute. *Clinical Guidelines on the Identification, Evaluation, and Treatment of Overweight and Obesity in Adults*. NIH Publication No. 98-4083. Bethesda, MD: National Institutes of Health, September 1998.

Pasanisi F, Contaldo F, de Simone G, Mancini M. Benefits of sustained moderate weight loss in obesity. *Nutr Metab Cardiovasc Dis*. 2001;11:401–6.

Trentham-Dietz A, Newcomb PA, Egan KM, Titus-Ernstoff L, Baron JA, Storer BE, Stampfer M, Willett WC. Weight change and risk of postmenopausal breast cancer (United States). Cancer Causes Control 2000;11:533–42.

U.S. Department of Health and Human Services. Centers for Disease Control and Prevention. Third National Health and Nutrition Examination (NHANES III), 1988–94. www.cdc.gov.

U.S. Department of Health and Human Services. The Surgeon General's Call to Action to Prevent and Decrease Overweight and Obesity. Rockville, MD: U.S. Department of Health and Human Services, Public Health Service, Office of the Surgeon General; 2001.

## Chapter 3: Is willpower the key to weight loss?

DelParigi A, Chen K, Salbe AD, Hill JO, Wing RR, Reiman EM, Tataranni PA. Persistence of abnormal neural responses to a meal in postobese individuals. *Int J Obes Relat Metab Disord* 2004;28:370–7.

Heshka S, Anderson JW, Atkinson RL, Greenway FL, Hill JO, Phinney SD, Kolotkin RL, Miller-Kovach K, Pi-Sunyer FX. Weight loss with self-help compared with a structured commercial program: a randomized trial. *JAMA* 2003;289:1792–8.

Institute of Medicine. *Weighing the Options. Criteria for Evaluating Weight-Management Programs*. Washington, DC: National Academy Press, 1995.

Lowe MR. "Dietary Restraint and Overeating." Chapter 16. www.psychology.drexel.edu/papers/dietaryrestraint.doc.

Prochaska JO, Norcross JC, Fowler JL, Follick MJ, Abrams DB. Attendance and outcome in a work site weight control program: processes and stages of change as process and predictor variables. *Addict Behav* 1992;17:35–45.

Provencher V, Drapeau V, Tremblay A, Despres JP, Bouchard C, Lemieux S. Quebec Family Study. Eating behaviours, dietary profile and body composition according to dieting history in men and women of the Quebec Family Study. *Br J Nutr* 2004;91:997–1004.

Smith CF, Williamson DA, Bray GA, Ryan DH. Flexible vs. rigid dieting strategies: relationship with adverse behavioral outcomes. *Appetite* 1999;32:295–305.

Wing RR, Hill JO. Successful weight loss maintenance. *Annu Rev Nutr* 2001;21:323–41.

Worcester MU, Stojcevski Z, Murphy B, Goble AJ. Long-term behavioral outcomes after attendance at a secondary prevention clinic for cardiac patients. *J Cardiopulm Rehab* 2003:23:423–5.

## Chapter 4: Should I focus mostly on exercise?

Andersen RE, Wadden TA, Bartlett SJ, Zemel B, Verde TJ, Franckowiak SC. Effects of lifestyle activity vs structured aerobic exercise in obese women: a randomized trial. *JAMA* 1999;281:335–40.

Centers for Disease Control and Prevention (CDC). Trends in intake of energy and macronutrients—United States, 1971–2000. *MMWR Morb Mortal Wkly Rep* 2004;53:80–2.

Egger GJ, Vogels N, Westerterp KR. Estimating historical changes in physical activity levels. *Med J Aust* 2001;175:635–6.

Enns CW, Goldman JD, Cook A. Trends in food consumption and nutrient intakes by adults: NFCS 1977–78, CSFII 1989–91, and CSFII 1994–95. *Family Economics and Nutrition Review*. www.barc.usda.gov/bhnrc/foodsurvey/pdf/Trends.pdf.

Fogelholm M, Kukkonen-Harjula K. Does physical activity prevent weight gain—a systematic review. *Obes Rev* 2000;1:95–111.

Jakicic JM, Polley BA, Wing RR. Accuracy of self-reported exercise and the relationship with weight loss in overweight women. *Med Sci Sports Exerc* 1998;30:634–8.

Jakicic JM, et al. American College of Sports Medicine Position Stand. Appropriate intervention strategies for weight loss and prevention of weight regain in adults. *Med Sci Sports Exerc* 2001;33:2145–56.

Klem ML, Wing RR, McGuire MT, Seagle HM, Hill, JO. A descriptive study of individuals successful at long-term maintenance of substantial weight loss. *Am J Clin Nutr* 1997;66:239–46.

Lissner L. Measuring food intake in studies of obesity. *Public Health Nutr* 2002; 5:889–92.

Marks B, Ward A, Castellani J, Fortlage L, Morris D, Puleo E, Webber L, Ahlquist L, Rippe J. The effect of a weight loss program on body composition changes in moderately obese women. *Med Sci Sports Exerc* 1991;23:S107.

Marks BL, Ward A, Morris DH, Castellani J, Rippe JM. Fat-free mass is maintained in women following a moderate diet and exercise program. *Med Sci Sports Exerc* 1995;27:1243–51.

National Heart, Lung, and Blood Institute. *Clinical Guidelines on the Identification, Evaluation, and Treatment of Overweight and Obesity in Adults.* NIH Publication No. 98-4083. Bethesda, MD: National Institutes of Health, September 1998.

Rippe JM, Price JM, Hess SA, Kline G, DeMers KA, Damitz S, Kreidieh I, Freedson P. Improved psychological well-being, quality of life, and health practices in moderately overweight women participating in a 12-week structured weight loss program. *Obes Res* 1998;6:208–18.

Saris WH. Fit, fat and fat free: the metabolic aspects of weight control. *Int J Obes Relat Metab Disord* 1998;S2:S15–21.

Schoeller DA, et al. How much physical activity is needed to minimize weight gain in previously obese women? *Am J Clin Nutr* 1997;66:551–6.

U.S. Department of Agriculture. Trends in Food and Nutrient Intakes by Adults. Continuing Survey of Food Intakes by Individuals (CSFII), 1994. 95. www.barc.usda.gov.

U.S. Department of Health and Human Services. *Healthy People 2010*, 2nd ed. *Understanding and Improving Health Objectives for Improving Health.* Washington, DC: Government Printing Office, 2000.

U.S. Surgeon General. *The Surgeon General's Call to Action to Prevent and Decrease Overweight and Obesity.* www.surgeongeneral.gov/topics/obesity/calltoaction/fact_whatcanyoudo.htm.

U.S. Surgeon General. *The Surgeon General's Report on Physical Activity and Health.* www.cdc.gov/nccdphp/sgr/sgr.htm.

## Chapter 5: What counts the most—fats, carbs, or calories?

American Diabetes Association. Nutrition principles and recommendations in diabetes. *Diabetes Care* 2004;27:S36.

Bravata DM, et al. Efficacy and safety of low-carbohydrate diets. *JAMA* 2003;289:1837–50.

Bray GA. Low-carbohydrate diets and realities of weight loss. *JAMA* 2003;289:1853–5.

de Lorgeril M, Salen P, Martin JL, Monjaud I, Boucher P, Mamelle N. Mediterranean dietary pattern in a randomized trial: prolonged survival and possible reduced cancer rate. *Arch Intern Med* 1998;158:1181–7.

de Lorgeril M, Salen P, Martin JL, Monjaud I, Delaye J, Mamelle N. Mediterranean diet, traditional risk factors, and the rate of cardiovascular complications after myocardial infarction: final report of the Lyon Diet Heart Study. *Circulation* 1999;99:779–85.

Drewnowski A. Intense sweeteners and the control of appetite. *Nutr Rev* 1995;53(1):1–7.

Enns CW, Goldman JD, Cook A. Trends in food and nutrient intakes by adults: NFCS 1977–78, CSFII 1989–91, and CSFII 1994–95. *Family Economics and Nutrition Review* 1997;10:2–15. www.barc.usda.gov/bhnrc/foodsurvey/pdf/Trends.pdf.

Foster GD, et al. A randomized trial of a low-carbohydrate diet for obesity. *N Engl J Med* 2003;348:2074–81.

Freedman MR, King J, Kennedy E. Popular diets: a scientific review. *Obes Res* 2001;9(supp. 1):1S–40S.

Golay A, et al. Similar weight loss with low- or high-carbohydrate diets. *Am J Clin Nutr* 1996;63:174–8.

Hill JO. "Lessons from Successful Losers: The National Weight Control Registry." Presentation, July 22, 2003.

Institute of Food Technologists. *What, When and Where Americans Eat in 2003*. www.ift.org.

Institute of Medicine. *Dietary Reference Intakes for Vitamin C, Vitamin E, Selenium, and Carotenoids*. Washington, DC: National Academy Press, 2000.

Institute of Medicine. *Dietary Reference Intakes for Energy, Carbohydrate, Fiber, Fat, Fatty Acids, Cholesterol, Protein, and Amino Acids*. Washington, DC: National Academy Press, 2002.

Kappagoda CT, Hyson DA, Amsterdam EA. Low-carbohydrate high-protein diets. *J Am Coll Cardiol* 2004;43:725–30.

Lowe ML, Thaw J, Miller-Kovach K. Long-term follow-up assessment of successful dieters in a commercial weight-loss program. *Int J Obes Relat Metab Disord* 2004;28(suppl 1):S29.

Mattes R. Effects of aspartame and sucrose on hunger and energy intake in humans. *Physiol Behav* 1990;47(6):1037–44.

McManus K, Antinoro L, Sacks F. A randomized controlled trial of a moderate-fat, low-energy diet compared with a low-fat, low-energy diet for weight loss in overweight adults. *Int J Obes Relat Metab Disord* 2001;25:1503–11.

Samaha FF, et al. A low-carbohydrate as compared with a low-fat diet in severe obesity. *N Engl J Med* 2003;2074–81.

St. Jeor ST, et al. AHA Science Advisory. Dietary protein and weight reduction. *Circulation* 2001;104:1869.

Stein K. High-protein, low-carbohydrate diets: Do they work? *J Am Diet Assoc* 2000;100:760–1.

Weinberg SL. The diet-heart hypothesis: a critique. *J Am Coll Cardiol* 2004;43:731–3.

Westman EC, et al. Effect of 6-month adherence to a very low carbohydrate diet program. *Am J Med* 2002;113:30–6.

Willett WC. Reduced-carbohydrate diets: no roll in weight management? *Ann Intern Med* 2004;140:836–7.

## Chapter 6: Do my genes or metabolism keep me from achieving sustainable weight loss?

Asbeck I, Mast M, Bierwag A, Westenhofer J, Acheson KJ, Muller MJ. Severe underreporting of energy intake in normal weight subjects: use of an appropriate standard and relation to restrained eating. *Public Health Nutr* 2002;5:683–90.

Buhl KM, Gallagher D, Hoy K, Matthews DE, Heymsfield SB. Unexplained disturbance in body weight regulation: diagnostic outcome assessed by doubly labeled water and body composition analyses in obese patients reporting low energy intakes. *J Am Diet Assoc* 1995;95:1393–400.

Bulik CM, Sullivan PF, Kendler KS. Genetic and environmental contributions to obesity and binge eating. *Int J Eat Disord* 2003;33:293–8.

Caan B, Coates A, Schaefer C, Finkler L, Sternfeld B, Corbett K. Women gain weight 1 year after smoking cessation while dietary intake temporarily increases. *J Am Diet Assoc* 1996;96:1150–5.

Damcott CM, Sack P, Shuldiner AR. The genetics of obesity. *Endocrinol Metab Clin North Am* 2003;32:761–86.

Filozof C, Fernandez Pinilla MC, Fernandez-Cruz A. Smoking cessation and weight gain. *Obes Rev* 2004;5:95–103.

Flegel KM, Carroll MD, Kuczmarski RJ, Johnson CL. Overweight and obesity in the United States: prevalence and trends, 1960–1994. *Int J Obes Relat Metab Disord* 1998;22:39–47.

Gavaler JS, Rosenblum E. Predictors of postmenopausal body mass index and waist hip ratio in the Oklahoma Postmenopausal Health Disparities Study. *J Am Coll Nutr* 2003;22:269–76.

Hainer V, Stunkard A, Kunesova M, Parizkova J, Stich V, Allison DB. A twin study of weight loss and metabolic efficiency. *Int J Obes Relat Metab Disord* 2001;25:533–7.

Horner NK, Patterson RE, Neuhouser ML, Lampe JW, Beresford SA, Prentice RL. Participant characteristics associated with errors in self-reported energy intake from the Women's Health Initiative food-frequency questionnaire. *Am J Clin Nutr* 2002;76:766–73.

John Hancock Center for Physical Activity and Nutrition. *Burning Calories Is Not an Exact Science.* www.nutrition.tufts.edu/research/jhcpan/consumers/burning_calories.html.

Jones A Jr, Shen W, St-Onge MP, Gallagher D, Heshka S, Wang Z, Heymsfield SB. Body-composition differences between African American and white women: relation to resting energy requirements. *Am J Clin Nutr* 2004;79:780–6.

Kawachi I, Troisi RJ, Rotnitzky AG, Coakley EH, Colditz GA. Can physical activity minimize weight gain in women after smoking cessation? *Am J Public Health* 1996;86:925–6.

Keller KL, Pietrobelli A, Must S, Faith MS. Genetics of eating and its relation to obesity. *Curr Atheroscler Rep* 2002;4:176–82.

Lafay L, Mennen L, Basdevant A, Charles MA, Borys JM, Eschwege E, Romon M. Does energy intake underreporting involve all kinds of food or only specific food items? Results from the Fleurbaix Laventie Ville Sante (FLVS) study. *Int J Obes Relat Metab Disord* 2000;24:1500–6.

National Heart, Lung, and Blood Institute. *Clinical Guidelines on the Identification, Evaluation, and Treatment of Overweight and Obesity in Adults.* NIH Publication No. 98-4083. Bethesda, MD: National Institutes of Health, September 1998.

Novotny JA, Rumpler WV, Riddick H, Hebert JR, Rhodes D, Judd JT, Baer DJ, McDowell M, Briefel R. Personality characteristics as predictors of underreporting of energy intake on 24-hour dietary recall interviews. *J Am Diet Assoc* 2003; 103:1146–51.

O'Toole ML, Sawicki MA, Artal R. Structured diet and physical activity prevent postpartum weight retention. *J Women's Health (Larchmt)* 2003;12:991–8.

Rooney BL, Schauberger CW. Excess pregnancy weight gain and long-term obesity: one decade later. *Obstet Gyn* 2002;100:245–52.

Simkin-Silverman LR, Wing RR, Boraz MA, Kuller LH. Lifestyle intervention can prevent weight gain during menopause: results from a 5-year randomized clinical trial. *Ann Behav Med* 2003;26:212–20.

Snijder MB, Kuyf BE, Deurenberg P. Effect of body build on the validity of predicted body fat from body mass index and bioelectrical impedance. *Ann Nutr Metab* 1999;43:277–85.

van den Brule F, Gaspard U. Body mass changes at menopause: impact of therapeutic strategies. *Rev Med Liege* 2003;58:734–40.

Walsh MC, Hunter GR, Sirikul B, Gower BA. Comparison of self-reported with objectively assessed energy expenditure in black and white women before and after weight loss. *Am J Clin Nutr* 2004;79:1013–9.

Weinsier RL, Hunter GR, Zuckerman PA, Darnell BE. Low resting and sleeping energy expenditure and fat use do not contribute to obesity in women. *Obes Res* 2003;11:937–44.

Zhu S, Heshka S, Wang Z, Shen W, Allison DB, Ross R, Heymsfield SB. Combination of BMI and waist circumference for identifying cardiovascular risk factors in whites. *Obes Res* 2004;12:633–45.

## Chapter 7: Is my metabolism affected by what, how, and when I eat?

Buchholz AC, Schoeller DA. Is a calorie a calorie? *Am J Clin Nutr* 2004;79:899S–906S.

Demling RH, DeSanti L. Effect of a hypocaloric diet, increased protein intake and resistance training on lean mass gains and fat mass loss in overweight police officers. *Ann Nutr Metab* 2000;44:21–9.

Farshchi HR, Taylor MA, Macdonald IA. Decreased thermic effect of food after an irregular compared with a regular meal pattern in healthy lean women. *Int J Obes Relat Metab Disord* 2004;28:653–60.

Golay A, Allaz AF, Ybarra J, Bianchi P, Saraiva S, Mensi N, Gomis R, de Tonnac N. Similar weight loss with low-energy food combining or balanced diets. *Int J Obes Relat Metab Disord* 2000; 24:492–6.

Gore SA, Foster JA, DiLillo VG, Kirk K, Smith West D. Television viewing and snacking. *Eat Behav* 2003;4:399–405.

Kovacs EM, Lejeune MP, Nijs I, Westerterp-Plantenga MS. Effects of green tea on weight maintenance after body-weight loss. *Br J Nutr* 2004;91:431–7.

Kruger J, Galuska DA, Serdula MK, Jones DA. Attempting to lose weight: specific practices among U.S. adults. *Am J Prev Med* 2004;26:402–6.

Laforgia J, Withers RT, Shipp NJ, Gore CJ. Comparison of energy expenditure elevations after submaximal and supramaximal running. *J Appl Physiol* 1997;82:661–6.

Lejeune MP, Kovacs EM, Westerterp-Plantenga MS. Effect of capsaicin on substrate oxidation and weight maintenance after modest body-weight loss in human subjects. *Br J Nutr* 2003;90:651–59.

Luscombe ND, Clifton PM, Noakes M, Farnsworth E, Wittert G. Effect of a high-protein, energy-restricted diet on weight loss and energy expenditure after weight stabilization in hyperinsulinemic subjects. *Int J Obes Relat Metab Disord* 2003;27:582–90.

Makris AP, Rush CR, Frederich RC, Kelly TH. Wake-promoting agents with different mechanisms of action: comparison of effects of modafinil and amphetamine on food intake and cardiovascular activity. *Appetite* 2004;42:185–95.

Mazzoni R, Mannucci E, Rizzello SM, Ricca V, Rotella CM. Failure of acupuncture in the treatment of obesity: a pilot study. *Eat Weight Disord* 1999;4:198–202.

Merikle PM, Skanes HE. Subliminal self-help audiotapes: a search for placebo effects. *J Appl Psychol* 1992;77:772–6.

Nordenberg T. The healing power of placebos. *FDA Consumer*. January–February 2000.

Sensi S, Capani F. Chronobiological aspects of weight loss in obesity: effects of different meal timing regimens. *Chronobiol Int* 1987;4:251–61.

Speakman JR, Selman C. Physical activity and resting metabolic rate. *Proc Nutr Soc* 2003;62:621–34.

Tai MM, Castillo P, Pi-Sunyer FX. Meal size and frequency: effect on the thermic effect of food. *Am J Clin Nutr* 1991;54:783–7.

Taylor E, Missik E, Hurley R, Hudak S, Logue E. Obesity treatment: broadening our perspective. *Am J Health Behav* 2004;28:242–9.

Weight-control Information Network. *Weight-loss and Nutrition Myths. How Much Do You Really Know?* NIH Publication No. 04-4561. March 2004. www.niddk.nih.gov/health/nutrit/pubs/myths/index.htm.

## Chapter 8: Does how I lose weight really matter?

Atkinson RL, Fuchs A, Pastors JG, Saunders JT. Combination of very-low-calorie diet and behavior modification in the treatment of obesity. *Am J Clin Nutr* 1992;56(suppl 1):199S–202S.

Blair SN, LaMonte MJ, Nichaman MZ. The evolution of physical activity recommendations: how much is enough? *Am J Clin Nutr* 2004;79:913S–20S.

Centers for Disease Control. National Center for Chronic Disease Prevention and Health Promotion. *Physical Activity*. www.cdc.gov/nccdphp/dnpa/physical/.

Gornall J, Villani RG. Short-term changes in body composition and metabolism with severe dieting and resistance exercise. *Int J Sport Nutr* 1996;6:285–94.

Institute of Medicine. *Weighing the Options. Criteria for Evaluating Weight-Management Programs*. Washington, DC: National Academy Press, 1995.

Institute of Medicine. *Dietary Reference for Intakes of Water, Potassium, Sodium, Chloride, and Sulfate*. Washington, DC: National Academy Press, 2004.

Kamrath RO, Plummer LJ, Sadur CN, Adler MA, Strader WJ, Young RL, Weinstein RL. Cholelithiasis in patients treated with a very-low-calorie diet. *Am J Clin Nutr* 1992;56(suppl 1):255S–7S.

Kreitzman SN, Coxon AY, Szaz KF. Glycogen storage: illusions of easy weight loss, excessive weight regain, and distortions in estimates of body composition. *Am J Clin Nutr* 1992;56(suppl 1):292S–3S.

Phelan S, Hill JO, Lang W, Dibello JR, Wing RR. Recovery from relapse among successful weight maintainers. *Am J Clin Nutr* 2003;78:1079–84.

Plodkowski RA, St Jeor ST. Medical nutrition therapy for the treatment of obesity. *Endocrinol Metab Clin North Am* 2003;32:935–65.

Shibata M, Nakamuta H, Abe S, Kume K, Yoshikawa I, Murata I, Otsuki M. Ischemic colitis caused by strict dieting in an 18-year-old female: report of a case. *Dis Colon Rectum* 2002;45:425–8.

St Jeor ST, Brunner RL, Harrington ME, Scott BJ, Daugherty SA, Cutter GR, Brownell KD, Dyer AR, Foreyt JP. A classification system to evaluate weight maintainers, gainers, and losers. *J Am Diet Assoc* 1997;97:481–8.

Thwaites BC, Bose M. Very low calorie diets and pre-fasting prolonged QT interval. A hidden potential danger. *West Indian Med J* 1992;41:169–71.

Wadden TA. Treatment of obesity by moderate and severe caloric restriction. Results of clinical research trials. *Ann Intern Med* 1993;119:688–93.

Westenhoefer J, Stunkard AJ, Pudel V. Validation of the flexible and rigid control dimensions of dietary restraint. *Int J Eat Disord* 1999;26:53–64.

## Chapter 9: Is there one right approach to weight loss?

American Heart Association. www.americanheart.org.

Baker RC, Kirschenbaum DS. Weight control during the holidays: highly consistent self-monitoring as a potentially useful coping mechanism. *Health Psychol* 1998;17:367–70.

Boutelle KN, Kirschenbaum DS. Further support for consistent self-monitoring as a vital component of successful weight control. *Obes Res* 1998;6:219–24.

Buchholz AC, Schoeller DA. Is a calorie a calorie? *Am J Clin Nutr* 2004;79:899S–906S.

Canetti L, Bachar E, Berry EM. Food and emotion. *Behav Processes* 2002;60:157–64.

Cho S, Dietrich M, Brown CJ, Clark CA, Block G. The effect of breakfast type on total daily energy intake and body mass index: results from the Third National Health and Nutrition Examination Survey (NHANES III). *J Am Coll Nutr* 2003;22(4): 296–302.

Daniel ES. "House Calls—Obesity treatment." Senior World Online. www.seniorworld.com/articles/a19991209135525.html.

Devitt AA, Mattes RD. Effects of food unit size and energy density on intake in humans. *Appetite* 2004;42:213–20.

Drewnowski A, Specter SE. Poverty and obesity: the role of energy density and energy costs. *Am J Clin Nutr* 2004;79:6–16.

Fedoroff I, Polivy J, Herman CP. The specificity of restrained versus unrestrained eaters' responses to food cues: general desire to eat, or craving for the cued food? *Appetite* 2003;41:7–13.

Gerstein DE, Woodward-Lopez G, Evans AE, Kelsey K, Drewnowski A. Clarifying concepts about macronutrients' effects on satiation and satiety. *J Am Diet Assoc* 2004;104:1151–3.

Howarth NC, Saltzman E, Roberts SB. Dietary fiber and weight regulation. *Nutr Rev* 2001;59:129–39.

Institute of Medicine. *Weighing the Options*. Washington, DC: National Academy Press, 1995.

Koh-Banerjee P, Rimm EB. Whole grain consumption and weight gain: a review of the epidemiological evidence, potential mechanisms and opportunities for future research. *Proc Nutr Soc* 2003;62:25–9.

Latner JD, Stunkard AJ, Wilson GT, Jackson ML, Zelitch DS, Labouvie E. Effective long-term treatment of obesity: a continuing care model. *Int J Obes Relat Metab Disord* 2000;24:893–8.

Mattfeldt-Beman MK, Corrigan SA, Stevens VJ, Sugars CP, Dalcin AT, Givi MJ, Copeland KC. Participants' evaluation of a weight-loss program. *J Am Diet Assoc* 1999;99:66–71.

"Methods for Voluntary Weight Loss and Control." NIH Technol Assess Statement Online Mar 30–Apr 1, 1992. Cited July 30, 2004.

National Arts Journalism Program at Columbia University."Best and Worst of Times: Best Books vs. Bestsellers in a Changing Business." www.najp.org/conferences/books/summary.html.

National Institutes of Health Weight-control Information Network. www.niddk.nih.gov/health/nutrit/pubs/choose.htm.

O'Neil PM. Assessing dietary intake in the management of obesity. *Obes Res* 2001;9(suppl 5):361S-6S; discussion 373S–4S.

Partnership for Healthy Weight Management. www.ftc.gov/bcp/conline/pubs/health/wgtloss.pdf.

Plodkowski RA, St Jeor ST. Medical nutrition therapy for the treatment of obesity. *Endocrinol Metab Clin North Am* 2003;32:935–65.

Rolls BJ, Ello-Martin JA, Tohill BC. What can intervention studies tell us about the relationship between fruit and vegetable consumption and weight management? *Nutr Rev* 2004;62:1–17.

Stubbs J, Ferres S, Horgan G. Energy density of foods: effects on energy intake. *Crit Rev Food Sci Nutr* 2000;40:481–515.

Stunkard AJ. Current views on obesity. *Am J Med* 1996;100(2):230–6.

Wing RR, Hill JO. Successful weight loss maintenance. *Annu Rev Nutr* 2001;21:323–41.

Wyatt HR, Grunwald GK, Mosca CL, Klem ML, Wing RR, Hill JO. Long-term weight loss and breakfast in subjects in the National Weight Control Registry. *Obes Res* 2002;10(2):78–82.

Yao M, Roberts SB. Dietary energy density and weight regulation. *Nutr Rev* 2001;59(8, Pt 1):247–58.

## Chapter 10: Is my weight problem just about me?

Andrews G. Intimate saboteurs. *Obes Surg* 1997;7:445–8.

Benton D. Role of parents in the determination of the food preferences of children and the development of obesity. *Int J Obes Relat Metab Disord* 2004;28:858–69.

Birch LL, Fisher JO. Development of eating behaviors among children and adolescents. *Pediatrics* 1998;101:539–49.

Black DR. Weight changes in a couples program: negative association of marital adjustment. *J Behav Ther Exp Psychiatry* 1988;19:103–11.

Black DR, Gleser LJ, Kooyers KJ. A meta-analytic evaluation of couples weight-loss programs. *Health Psychol* 1990;9:330–47.

Bloch KV, Klein CH, de Souza e Silva NA, Nogueira Ada R, Salis LH. Socioeconomic aspects of spousal concordance for hypertension, obesity, and smoking in a community of Rio de Janeiro, Brazil. *Arq Bras Cardiol* 2003;80:171–8,179–86.

Burke V, Mori TA, Giangiulio N, Gillam HF, Beilin LJ, Houghton S, Cutt HE, Mansour J, Wilson A. An innovative program for changing health behaviours. *Asia Pac J Clin Nutr* 2002;11(suppl 3):S586–97.

Casey R, Rozin P. Changing children's food preferences: parent opinions. *Appetite* 1989;12:171–82.

Centers for Disease Control. "Obesity Costs States Billions in Medical Expenses." Press release, January 21, 2004. www.cdc.gov/od/oc/media/pressrel/r040121.htm.

Epstein LH. Exercise in the treatment of childhood obesity. *Int J Obes Relat Metab Disord* 1995;19(suppl 4):S117–21.

Finkelstein EA, Fiebelkorn IC, Wang G. National medical spending attributable to overweight and obesity: how much, and who's paying? *Health Affairs*, Web exclusive, May 14, 2003.

Foreyt JP, Ramirez AG, Cousins JH. Cuidando El Corazon—a weight-reduction intervention for Mexican Americans. *Am J Clin Nutr* 1991;53(suppl 6):1639S–41S.

Forster JL, Jeffery RW. Gender differences related to weight history, eating patterns, efficacy expectations, self-esteem, and weight loss among participants in a weight reduction program. *Addict Behav* 1986;11:141–7.

Heshka S, Anderson JW, Atkinson RL, Greenway FL, Hill JO, Phinney SD, Kolotkin RL, Miller-Kovach K, Pi-Sunyer FX. Weight loss with self-help compared with a structured commercial program: a randomized trial. *JAMA* 2003;289:1792–8.

Jeffery RW, Rick AM. Cross-sectional and longitudinal associations between body mass index and marriage-related factors. *Obes Res* 2002;10:809–15.

Kahn HS, Williamson DF. The contributions of income, education and changing marital status to weight change among US men. *Int J Obes Relat Metab Disord* 1990;14:1057–68.

Karlsson J, Taft C, Sjostrom L, Torgerson JS, Sullivan M. Psychosocial functioning in the obese before and after weight reduction: construct validity and responsiveness of the Obesity-related Problems Scale. *Int J Obes Relat Metab Disord* 2003;27:617–30.

Kratt P, Reynolds K, Shewchuk R. The role of availability as a moderator of family fruit and vegetable consumption. *Health Educ Behav* 2000;27:471–82.

Marchesini G, Solaroli E, Baraldi L, Natale S, Migliorini S, Visani F, Forlani G, Melchionda N. Health-related quality of life in obesity: the role of eating behaviour. *Diabetes Nutr Metab* 2000;13:156–64.

Marchesini G, Natale S, Chierici S, Manini R, Besteghi L, Di Domizio S, Sartini A, Pasqui F, Baraldi L, Forlani G, Melchionda N. Effects of cognitive-behavioural therapy on health-related quality of life in obese subjects with and without binge eating disorder. *Int J Obes Relat Metab Disord* 2002;26:1261–7.

Rippe JM, Price JM, Hess SA, Kline G, DeMers KA, Damitz S, Kreidieh I, Freedson P. Improved psychological well-being, quality of life, and health practices in moderately overweight women participating in a 12-week structured weight loss program. *Obes Res* 1998;6:208–18.

Roberts RE, Strawbridge WJ, Deleger S, Kaplan GA. Are the fat more jolly? *Ann Behav Med* 2002;24:169–80.

Sobal J, Rauschenbach B, Frongillo EA. Marital status changes and body weight changes: a US longitudinal analysis. *Soc Sci Med* 2003;56:1543–55.

Wade TD, Lowes J. Variables associated with disturbed eating habits and overvalued ideas about the personal implications of body shape and weight in a female adolescent population. *Int J Eat Disord* 2002;32:39–45.

Wardle J, Guthrie C, Sanderson S, Birch L, Plomin R. Food and activity preferences in children of lean and obese parents. *Int J Obes Relat Metab Disord* 2001;25:971–7.

White E, Hurlich M, Thompson RS, Woods MN, Henderson MM, Urban N, Kristal A. Dietary changes among husbands of participants in a low-fat dietary intervention. *Am J Prev Med* 1991;7:319–25.

Wing RR, Jeffery RW. Benefits of recruiting participants with friends and increasing social support for weight loss and maintenance. *J Consult Clin Psychol* 1999;67: 132–8.

Wolfe WA. A review: maximizing social support—a neglected strategy for improving weight management with African-American women. *Ethn Dis* 2004;14:212–8.

# Index